Getting Health Economics into Practice

Edited by
David Kernick

Radcliffe Medical Press

Radcliffe Medical Press Ltd
18 Marcham Road
Abingdon
Oxon OX14 1AA
United Kingdom

www.radcliffe-oxford.com
The Radcliffe Medical Press electronic catalogue and online ordering facility.
Direct sales to anywhere in the world.

British Library Cataloguing in Publication Data

A catalogue record for this book is available from the British Library.

ISBN 1 85775 575 8

Typeset by Aarontype Ltd, Easton, Bristol
Printed and bound by TJ International Ltd, Padstow, Cornwall

Contents

About this book

Who is it directed at?

All those who are involved in the planning, commissioning and delivery of healthcare.

What are its aims?

- To illuminate the concepts and principles that health economics can offer decision makers at all levels.
- To address the dissonance between health economic rhetoric and the reality of the healthcare environment.

Where is it coming from?

This book is orchestrated from the 'swampy lowlands' of healthcare where life is not always about cosy certainties like evidence-based medicine and the results of economic studies. It is written in a way that is accessible to end users of economic information.

Who is the editor?

David Kernick started life as a chemical engineer but has been a full time general practitioner for 19 years.

As Lead Research General Practitioner in a large group practice that receives funding from the NHS Research & Development Directorate, he is interested in addressing the gap between health economic theory and the practical realities of healthcare decision making.

As Medical Officer to Exeter City Football Club he supports their eternal struggle to stay in the Third Division of the Football League.

He has no qualifications or training in health economics.

List of contributors

John Appleby
Director
Health Systems Programme
The King's Fund
London

Joanna Coast
Senior Lecturer in Health Economics
Department of Social Medicine
University of Bristol

Huw Davies
Reader in Healthcare Policy & Management
University of St Andrews

Martyn Evans
Professor of Humanities in Medicine
University of Durham
and
Principal, John Snow College
University of Durham

Shelley Farrar
Research Fellow
Health Economics Research Unit
University of Aberdeen

David Kernick
General Practitioner
St Thomas Medical Group
Exeter

Martin Knapp
Professor of Social Policy
PSSRU
London School of Economics, Health & Social Care

Donald Light
Professor of Comparative Health Care Systems
University of Medicine & Dentistry of New Jersey

Russell Mannion
Senior Research Fellow
Centre for Health Economics
University of York

Alan Maynard
Professor of Health Economics
Health Economics Consortium
University of York

Ruth McDonald
NHS/PPP Research Fellow
Department of Applied Social Science
University of Manchester

Rebecca Mears
Research Fellow
Department of Public Health & Epidemiology
University of Birmingham

Gill Morgan
Chief Executive
NHS Confederation

Ann Netten
Director and Senior Research Fellow
PSSRU
University of Kent

Christopher Newdick
Reader
Department of Law
University of Reading

Charles Normand
Professor of Health Economics
Head of Department of Epidemiology & Population Health
London School of Hygiene & Tropical Medicine

Denis Pereira Gray
Emeritus Professor of General Practice
Institute of General Practice/SaNDNet
School of Sport & Health Sciences
University of Exeter

Caroline Reeves
Research Assistant
Health Economics Research Unit
University of Aberdeen

Ray Robinson
Professor of Health Policy
The London School of Economics

Mandy Ryan
Senior Fellow and Reader in Health Economics
Health Economics Research Unit
University of Aberdeen

Anthony Scott
Programme Director and Senior Research Fellow
Health Economics Research Unit
University of Aberdeen

Rod Taylor
Senior Lecturer
Department of Public Health & Epidemiology
University of Birmingham

Tom Walley
Professor of Pharmacology & Therapeutics
National Prescribing Centre
Liverpool

Paul Webley
Professor of Economic Psychology
School of Psychology
University of Exeter

Adrian White
Senior Lecturer
Department of Complementary Medicine
University of Exeter

Prologue

Better to be vaguely right than precisely wrong

Fifty years ago medicine was straightforward. Doctors had limited therapeutic options and patients did as they were told. Now, an array of medical interventions is putting increasing pressure on limited resources, patients are questioning everything and doctors are uncertain of their role. Medicine has been transformed into healthcare, a multiplicity of disciplines that includes management science, epidemiology, psychology and sociology.

Health economists have been the latest addition to the melting pot, applying economic theory to problems in healthcare. Thirty years ago the new discipline set off with high hopes to offer important insights at all levels of decision making but unfortunately, the resulting programme has not formed a homogeneous amalgam with other healthcare perspectives. Policy makers and practitioners continue in their struggle to mediate between the resource requirements of public policies and the demands of patients in an environment characterised by complexity, value conflict, paradox and limited room for manoeuvre.

The reason for the dissonance between health economic rhetoric and health service reality is demonstrated by the words of Professor Alan Williams, one of the founding fathers of the subject. In the early 1970s, when health economics was branching out from its parent discipline, he suggested to his colleagues that 'Until we are able to explain to medics and managers in rather simple terms what we are at, we had better keep such studies strictly within the family.' Health economic theory was to be canonised in ivory towers uncontaminated by the realities of the emerging healthcare environment. The result was the development of inaccessible technical frameworks that bore little resemblance to the practical requirements of end users. It appeared that the primary concern of health economists was to be an attempt to force reality into their disciplinary framework rather than the more logical converse.

More recently, health economists have come in from the cold and begun to work with decision makers. Their messages of scarcity, sacrifice and the need for explicit resource allocation decisions have not always received a warm welcome, but health economists stress that they have not created the conditions from which the need for rationing arises. Rather, by offering methods for explicit prioritisation of healthcare, they see themselves as part of the solution.

The main aim of this book is to present the concepts and insights that health economics has to offer in a way that is accessible to healthcare decision makers at all levels. Its secondary aim is to highlight the gap between health economic rhetoric and the practical realities of health service life and the need to develop a discourse between health economists, healthcare managers, practitioners and patients.

Previous health economics texts for decision makers have been written from the academic 'sunny uplands'. Worthy but dull, the difficult realities of change are largely overlooked. This book is orchestrated from the 'swampy lowlands'. The author is a full-time general practitioner involved in a number of aspects of primary care organisation and research but with no formal training in health economics. This qualification offers a number of advantages: as a full time GP, the privilege of no academic constraint; as a generalist, a recognition that new knowledge can only arise from open conversation between different disciplines, not increasing demarcation between them; as a practitioner, an ability to live with paradox; as a health economics novice, insights into how the subject can be presented in a way that is accessible; with the experience of delivering and organising primary care, an appreciation of the decision-making frameworks that are required in the real world.

Hopefully, this book represents a genuine bottom-up attempt to get health economics into practice. Any errors are the responsibility of the editor alone. I merely refer to the economist John Maynard Keynes who, in a statement that health economists would do well to heed, claimed that it was 'better to be vaguely right than precisely wrong'.

Section 1

Getting to grips with the basics

The first section of this book lays out the basic framework of health economics for those who have no knowledge of the subject, introducing some basic concepts and principles.

Health economics applies economic theory to problems in healthcare and, like its parent discipline it has two distinct branches. One uses economic theory to understand how health systems work and how they can be configured to operate more effectively. The other uses economic theory to facilitate decisions on how to allocate limited resources efficiently between different healthcare interventions. Chapter 1 offers a brief introduction to economic theory and an overview of these two divisions, exploring how they can help facilitate decisions at all levels of healthcare planning and delivery. It also demonstrates how health economists are 'wired-up' to look at the world.

In Chapter 2, Anthony Scott addresses the first branch of health economics and explores how economic theory can explain and predict how health systems work and offers insights into how healthcare can be delivered. The starting point of any economic analysis is the assumption that a competitive market is the most efficient way to distribute limited resources. The problems of applying this model to healthcare are well recognised, but by using regulation and alternatives to markets, some of the desirable features of perfectly competitive markets can be replicated.

Of most interest to practitioners and healthcare managers will be the second branch of health economics. Economic evaluation aims to offer a framework within which the costs and benefits of alternative healthcare interventions can be compared. In Chapter 3, Ruth McDonald and I discuss in a little more detail the economic evaluation that forms the core of this book and provides the bulk of health economists' work.

CHAPTER 1

An introduction to health economics

David Kernick

This chapter outlines the basic principles of health economics and describes its context within the spectrum of healthcare decision making.

Key points
- Health economics is a subdiscipline of economics and is exerting an increasing impact on decisions in healthcare at every level.
- There are two distinct branches of economics and this distinction is carried through into health economics. One uses economic theory to explain and predict the operation of the health system. The other uses theory to facilitate decision making from a perspective of making the most efficient use of limited resources.
- Economic theory takes as its starting point the thesis that the most efficient way to distribute resources is using a market where individuals act rationally to maximise their satisfaction.
- The difficulties of applying this model to healthcare is well recognised, but its importance is that it provides useful insights into how healthcare can be organised and financed and it can provide a framework to address a broad range of issues in an explicit and consistent manner.
- Other inputs enter the decision-making process in healthcare such as equity and public opinion. These considerations can conflict with efficiency.
- Health economics has been slow to be adopted in practice due to a gap between health economic theory and the conflicting directives and pragmatic requirements of policy makers, managers and practitioners.

Chapter sections
- What is health economics?
- What drives health economists?

- What do health economists get up to?
- Conclusion

What is health economics?

Health economics is the discipline of economics applied to the topic of health. Broadly defined, economics concerns how society allocates its resources among alternative uses. Scarcity of these resources provides the foundation of economic theory and from this starting point three basic questions arise.

- What goods and services shall we produce?
- How shall we produce them?
- Who shall receive them?

Thirty years ago there were limited options for doctors making treatment choices and patients did as they were told. Any values that contributed to the decision-making process were implicit and determined by the physician. However, against a background of limited healthcare resources, an empowered consumer and an increasing array of intervention options, there is a need for decisions to be taken more openly and fairly.

Health economics offers an explicit explanatory and decision-making model based on the underlying value of efficiency. This approach ensures that goods and services are allocated in a way that maximises the welfare of the community. It is not the only approach to decision making but it is an important one.

The basic economic model

We need to make sense of the world and act. We do so using models that help us to see patterns in our environment. We create reality around 'bundles of related assumptions', conceptual lenses through which we view the world. All models are approximations but they can often be useful. Models help us with four basic questions.

- What does happen?
- What will happen?
- What would we like to happen? (For this stage, objectives need to be defined and values made explicit so that judgements can be made about what is right or wrong.)
- How can we make it happen using insights from our model?

The fundamental starting point of economic theory is that the best way of distributing society's limited resources is using the model of a competitive market where decisions are determined by independent consumers and producers using signals in the form of prices regulated by the interplay of supply and demand. Economics can be distinguished from other social sciences by the belief that behaviour can be explained by assuming that individuals have stable, well-defined preferences and make rational choices consistent with those preferences to maximise their own well being. These assumptions are known as the 'neo-classical' economic model. Although there are other economic frameworks, it is the most important one and the starting point for health economics. Box 1.1 outlines this economic model.

Box 1.1: The basic economic model upon which health economics is constructed. The model gives a predictive or explanatory framework (sometimes known as positive economics) – if certain actions are taken, certain results will follow and a prescriptive framework (sometimes known as normative economics) to facilitate decision making

- Resources are scarce and sacrifice is inevitable.
- The best way of distributing society's limited resources is using the model of a competitive market where decisions are determined by independent consumers and producers using signals in the form of prices regulated by the interplay of supply and demand.
- Each individual has preferences regarding the outputs of any given economic activity that can be ranked by priority and assigned utilities – quantitative measures of their ranking.
- People act as individuals and act so as to maximise their satisfaction or utility.
- The well being of society is reflected in the sum of the utilities of its individual citizens.

The difficulties of applying market theories to health are well recognised.

- There may be an uncertain relationship between the consumption of healthcare and health.
- Consumers do not have accurate information to allow them to make choices about their consumption of healthcare.
- There may be a reliance on clinicians to make choices on behalf of their patients, but these same clinicians as suppliers may have vested interests such as financial incentives.

- Consumers are not independent of each other's actions. Often, one individual's consumption of healthcare (e.g. immunisation) impacts on the health of others in the community.

The importance of the economic model is that it provides useful insights into how healthcare can be organised and financed, and provides a framework to address a broad range of issues in an explicit and consistent manner.

The two branches of health economics – descriptive and prescriptive

There are two distinct branches of economics that arise from the above economic model, and this distinction is carried through into health economics. The first branch of economics uses economic theory to explain and predict the operation of the economic system. This is referred to as positive or explanatory economics. The greater part of this book concerns itself with the second branch of economics that is of most relevance to decision makers. This branch is known as normative or welfare economics and uses economics to facilitate decision making from the perspective of making the most efficient use of limited resources. The practical expression of this search for efficiency in healthcare is the conduct of economic evaluation. This exercise offers a framework for measuring, valuing and comparing the costs (negative consequences) and benefits (positive consequences) of different healthcare interventions.

What drives health economists?

Underlying value systems

All choices depend to some extent on the value systems of decision makers. Clinicians have traditionally operated as advocates of the individual patient and have placed the highest value on patient well being irrespective of cost. In contrast, health economists adopt a value system directed by the most efficient use of resources from the perspective of society as a whole. However, this approach ignores the equity or fairness dimension of resource allocation. For example, it is generally agreed that patients should be treated equally irrespective of age, sex or socioeconomic status and those with greater need should receive preferential treatment. The principles of equity and their relationship with health economics are considered in more detail in Chapters 19 and 22. However, there are further problems.

A central tenant of government policy has been to involve the public in healthcare decision making. However, what consumers think, say and do is often very different. Insights from cognitive psychology demonstrate that the way that we make decisions is very different from the assumptions of economic theory. These problems are visited in Chapter 28.

In many cases, the inputs into decision making of efficiency, equity and public opinion are not compatible. For example, targeting health promotion at low-income smokers is equitable but not efficient compared with targeting higher socioeconomic groups. Investing resources in the care of very low birth weight babies has high levels of public support but is not efficient in terms of cost for each year of life saved. Many decisions will require a value judgement to weigh these different inputs.

Finally, even though an intervention may satisfy all the above criteria it may not be affordable. For example, lowering the cholesterol level of patients who have an annual risk of a cardiovascular event of 1.5% a year is an efficient use

Table 1.1:   Differences between accountants and health economists

Accountants	Health economists
• Interested only in monitoring finance, balancing budgets, focusing on cost control/containment	• Interested in defining and measuring a much broader range of costs which include those that are often not easy to measure (e.g. costs due to loss of work time, costs of suffering or loss of life)
• More interested in sources of finance and accuracy of financial estimates than in valuing the health implications of financial decisions (i.e. accountants are interested in valuing financial implications but only in terms of money, not benefits foregone)	• Stress the importance of valuing costs in terms of their lost opportunity (i.e. cost as sacrifice or what has to be gone without rather than just financial expenditure)
• Not interested in behavioural frameworks	• Stress the importance of scarcity, sacrifice and maximising utility or well being for understanding human behaviour
• Outcomes or health benefits of expenditure are of no interest	• Always relate resource use to resultant outcomes
• Accountants drive BMWs	• Health economists only drive BMWs if they work for the pharmaceutical industry

of resources in terms of cost for each year of life saved, is equitable and receives high levels of public support. Alas, it would consume 75% of the primary care drug budget![1]

How are health economists wired up?

Health economists are hard-wired to the fundamental model of a market and derivations of it as a basis for description and prescription. Their emphasis is on explicit and technical solutions. An economist has been described as one who 'by training thinks of himself as the guardian of rationality, the ascriber of rationality to others and the prescriber of rationality to the social world'.[2]

A common misconception is that health economists are like accountants – interested only in financial expenditure but with less imagination. Accountants have been compared with health economists to illuminate some important characteristics (Table 1.1).

What do health economists get up to?

Figure 1.1 shows a simple model of the generation of health. Society's resources are invested into a number of systems that address individual and population needs (e.g. education, sanitation, nutrition, healthcare) and as a result, health is maintained or improved. Healthcare is an important input but it is not the only one. (It has been estimated that of the 30-year increase in life expectancy witnessed in the twentieth century, medical interventions have contributed only five years[3] and the best estimates are that health services influence only 10% of the standard indices for measuring health.)

Health economists are interested in this process at a number of levels.

- What is health and how do we put a value on it?
- What influences health other than healthcare?
- What influences the demand for healthcare and healthcare seeking behaviour?
- What influences the supply of healthcare? (The behaviour of doctors and healthcare providers.)
- Alternative ways of production and delivery of healthcare.
- Planning, budgeting and monitoring of healthcare.
- Economic evaluation – relating the costs and benefits of alternative ways of delivering healthcare.

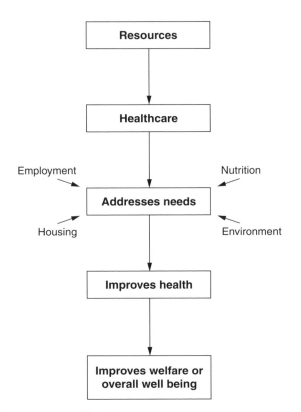

Figure 1.1: The generation of health.

Although we will meet all of these elements, it is economic evaluation that provides the bulk of health economists' work, is of most relevance to managers and practitioners and which forms the core of this book.

Conclusion

This chapter has set the context for health economics and its input into decision making. Against a background of increasing demands on limited healthcare resources, the emphasis is on providing an explicit and rational framework to facilitate healthcare choices from a perspective of efficiency. This seeks to maximise the population's health, but does not guide resource decisions when the perspective of equity or fairness is considered.

However, healthcare is not a machine that can be engineered towards defined objectives. It is often a complex environment of uncertain goals, historical precedent and limited room for manoeuvre. The dissonance between the economists' view of the world and the pragmatic requirements of healthcare providers and managers is a theme that runs throughout this book.

We now move on to explore in more detail the first major branch of health economics – positive or explanatory economics. The next chapter shows how economic theory can offer a framework to understand how healthcare systems work.

References

1   Pickin D, McCabe C, Ramsey L *et al*. (1999) Cost effectiveness of statin treatment related to the risk of coronary heart disease and cost of drug treatment. *Heart*. **82:** 325–32.
2   Arrow KJ (1974) In: L Tancredi (ed.) *Government Decision Making and the Preciousness of Life: ethics of healthcare*. National Academy of Sciences, Washington DC, Washington.
3   Bunker J and Frazier F (1994) Improving health measurement: effects of health and medical care. *Milbank Quarterly*. **72(2):** 225–58.

CHAPTER 2

Understanding healthcare delivery: the economic contribution

Anthony Scott

Positive or explanatory economics uses economic theory to explain and predict how the health system works. The delivery of healthcare using markets is the starting point of an economic analysis offering a framework to understand healthcare systems. This chapter considers how the real world differs from the ideal economic model and the insights that are obtained from such an approach.

Key points
- The delivery of healthcare using 'perfect' markets is the starting point of an economic analysis of the healthcare system.
- However, many assumptions underlying perfect markets do not apply in 'real world' healthcare systems.
- Understanding the differences between 'real world' health systems and perfect markets can offer insights into how healthcare delivery can be more efficient and equitable.
- By using regulation and alternatives to markets, some of the desirable features of perfectly competitive markets can be replicated.

Chapter sections
- **Introduction**
- **Causes of market failure and options for healthcare delivery**
- **Conclusion**

Introduction

The nature of healthcare delivery is complex and understanding it is crucial if healthcare systems are to be organised and financed in ways that meet society's objectives. The reform of healthcare delivery is constantly on the policy agenda as the search for improved healthcare systems continues. Reforms are usually focused on the scope, organisation and funding of the many different types of healthcare organisations. Reform also usually involves altering the relationships between healthcare organisations. At one extreme, such relationships involve 'arms-length' market transactions governed by explicit contracts and involving competition (the intention of the NHS internal market), and at the other extreme involve the vertical integration of healthcare organisations and reliance on cooperation and coordination. Organisations (and individuals within them) are also subject to varying degrees of performance management and monitoring.

Economic theory provides crucial insights into the workings of healthcare systems (and using this theory is necessary to 'get health economics into practice'). The delivery of healthcare using markets is the analytical starting point of the economist. This is not to say that economic theory is the 'right' theory to apply in healthcare, nor is it always applicable in healthcare – no single theory is 'right' or applicable. However, the value of economic theory is that it provides a framework that can be used to address a broad set of issues in a consistent and logical manner.

With respect to the analysis of healthcare delivery, the theoretical models of perfectly competitive markets and welfare economics are relevant starting points. Given the assumptions of these models, producers will produce goods and services at least cost (production efficiency), consumers will maximise utility given the resources they have (consumption efficiency), and society will maximise welfare given the existing distribution of resources (allocative or 'pareto' efficiency) (Box 2.1). In other words, everybody has maximised their

---

Box 2.1:   The basic model of a perfectly competitive market which is used as the starting point or the application of economic theory to health systems

- Producers will produce goods and services at least cost.
- Consumers will maximise their utility or well being given their available resources.
- Society will maximise its welfare given the existing distribution of resources.

utility (happiness or satisfaction) given the resources available, and it is not possible to make someone better off without making someone else worse off.

However, these utopian outcomes are confined to this model and do not occur in the real world. Many economists do not think that a perfect market can exist in practice due to its restrictive assumptions and the fact that it is a theoretical concept. Because of these assumptions, the models can be easily criticised as being unrealistic and, therefore, not relevant. However, the value of the perfectly competitive model is through comparing its assumptions to what happens in the real world. This enables analysts to explain the reasons why healthcare systems are organised and financed as they are, and suggests ways that efficiency and equity can be improved by changing the way healthcare is delivered. By using regulation and alternatives to markets, some of the desirable features of perfectly competitive markets can be replicated.

The aim of this chapter is to highlight the main economic issues concerned with healthcare delivery. The reasons why healthcare is delivered and financed in specific ways is examined by discussing the consequences of market failure in healthcare. A range of different methods of healthcare delivery is suggested in an attempt to address the problems caused by market failure.

Causes of market failure and options for healthcare delivery

Economic theory states that the ideal way to deliver any goods or services (including healthcare) is through a perfectly competitive market. However, most of the assumptions of the perfectly competitive model do not apply in healthcare. Compared to markets for most other goods and services, the inapplicability of the assumptions of the perfectly competitive model to healthcare is extensive, and provides powerful reasons why healthcare resources should not be allocated using unfettered market forces. These issues were first raised in the classic paper by Arrow,[1] and deal with three main assumptions of the economic model:

- certainty
- absence of externalities
- consumers having the same information as producers (symmetry of information).

The relationships between these assumptions and the system of healthcare delivery are shown in Table 2.1, and discussed below.

Table 2.1:   Links between market failure and healthcare delivery

Problems with the application of the economic model to healthcare	Implications	Solutions
• Uncertainty leading to the need to share risk through insurance (public or private)	• Dangers of monopoly provision of insurance due to diseconomies of small scale insurers • Adverse selection of risk by insurers • Lack of financial responsibility of consumers and producers (moral hazard)	• Public insurance • 100% coverage • Risk-adjusted private insurance • Budgets and payment systems for healthcare providers • User charges
• Externalities – spillovers of people's actions that affect a third party	• Inequity	• Public funding
• Asymmetry of information between consumers and suppliers of healthcare	• Supplier-induced demand	• Licensure, regulation and performance of providers • Payment systems • Doctor–patient communication

Uncertainty and the nature of healthcare insurance

The first reason why markets fail is the existence of uncertainty. As most people are uncertain about when they will use healthcare, how much they will use and how much it will cost, the response to this is to insure against these risks. A regular premium is paid to an insurance company that pools the risks of individual members. In return, the insurance company meets the cost of claims made by individuals who fall ill, under the terms of the insurance policy. Insurance can be provided by private insurance companies or, in the case of healthcare, by government. Premiums can be paid by individuals, their employer or through taxation. Premiums are comprised of expected healthcare expenditure and administrative costs. The former may be 'risk adjusted' and related to indicators of an individual's future risk of consuming healthcare (e.g. age, sex, previous health status) or may be 'community rated' where an average premium is set for everybody who is insured. There are three main reasons why most healthcare systems are not dominated by private insurance markets.

Diseconomies of small scale

The fixed costs of administration and marketing in private insurance companies are distributed among policy holders. Small companies will, therefore, have higher fixed costs per policy holder, thus increasing the premium compared to companies with a large number of policy holders who will be able to offer lower premiums. Small companies are therefore more likely to go out of business, as their relatively high premiums (compared to larger companies) mean that people are not insuring with them. This may lead to mergers and the existence of several large private insurance companies. The monopolistic nature of such a market may lead to potential exploitation of consumers because of the lack of competition that would otherwise keep premiums low. Diseconomies of small scale or monopolistic private insurance companies will keep premiums high. The key to this is that high premiums mean that many people do not insure, and these are most likely to be those least able to afford it as well as those most in need of healthcare.

Solutions – public insurance

Depending on the strength of preferences for equity (i.e. it may be considered unfair that people are not covered), this argument provides a justification for publicly provided insurance. This may involve collecting premiums through general taxation, or other means such as through systems of social insurance where administrative costs per insured person would be low. It may also involve insurance coverage for the whole population or for specific groups of the population who would not otherwise be covered.

Lack of financial responsibility by patients or doctors ('moral hazard')

The second reason why health systems are not dominated by private insurance is that neither patients nor doctors incur costs when they consume (or provide) healthcare, as these are reimbursed by the insurer. This is known as consumer and producer moral hazard. Consumer moral hazard is when patients may be more likely to visit the doctor if each visit is free to them, and perhaps less likely to adopt healthier lifestyles if they know that in the event of illness they will be cared for. This increases the consumption of healthcare, thus increasing costs, which leads to increased premiums and fewer people buying insurance. Again, the private insurance market may 'fail' because of the inability to control costs. Provider moral hazard is when healthcare providers do not face the costs of their decisions when recommending treatments for patients, as the insurance company will reimburse them for their time and any treatment recommendations (e.g. referrals and prescribing). Provider moral hazard is particularly problematic where doctors are paid by fee-for-service (FFS).

Solutions to consumer moral hazard – user charges

The main response to consumer moral hazard is to have user charges, where patients face some price when they consume healthcare. These are argued to limit the 'frivolous' demand caused by zero prices. Although there is strong evidence suggesting that user charges do reduce demand, there are many reasons why user charges may not be compatible with other health system goals. One of the strongest arguments, which is supported by some evidence, is that those least able to pay (and also the most in need of healthcare) would be deterred from using healthcare. As patients have little information about the relationship between healthcare and health status, they cannot judge whether their demand for healthcare is 'frivolous' or not. User charges may, therefore, deter those in need as well as the 'worried well'. Reducing demand also reduces demand for doctors' services and doctors' incomes. Depending on the way doctors are paid, doctors may, consequently, induce demand to maintain their incomes, which also increases costs. The result may be that the same amount is spent on healthcare, but would be targeted on the less needy, thus reducing efficiency and equity. The debate and evidence on the effects of user charges is extensive.[2]

Solutions to provider moral hazard – budgets and payment systems

The main response to provider moral hazard has been to make healthcare providers more aware of the costs of their actions by providing them with budgets or by paying them differently. Other responses have included ways of independently reviewing doctors' decisions, including utilisation review and clinical guidelines (although these have had less to do with costs).

Doctors have been given budgets in the UK through GP fundholding (abolished in 1997, although GPs continue to hold prescribing budgets and have some influence on budgets held by primary care groups), and through various budgetary incentives in health maintenance organisations (HMOs) in the USA. There is now a perception (with some evidence) that GP fundholding did not 'work', although the definition of success was never clear. Any cost savings were usually 'one-off', GPs inflated their activity before the scheme started in order to secure larger budgets and the effects of the scheme on patients' health status were never evaluated.[3] The scheme was also perceived as having adverse effects on equity of access, as GP fundholders could negotiate better deals with hospitals with respect to waiting times and other factors, and so discriminated against patients of non-GP fundholding practices.[4] However, this was related more to the voluntary nature of the scheme than the effect of fundholding *per se*.

Budgetary incentives in HMOs were much stronger relative to GP fundholding, in that surpluses could be retained by doctors as their own income, and financial penalties were incurred if they went over budget.[5] Although there is evidence that these 'managed care' arrangements (including budgets and salaried and captitation payment for doctors, rather than FFS) have reduced healthcare utilisation, there is mixed evidence of their effect on overall healthcare costs and on patients' health outcomes.[6,7]

Hospital payment systems are also important as potential solutions to provider moral hazard. Retrospective payments (based on the total cost of past activity) do not encourage cost consciousness and may encourage providers to maximise their budgets, unless budgets are capped in some way. Prospective payment is argued to reduce these incentives as hospitals are paid fees that are based on each patient's illness and treatment. Each patient is classified into a diagnosis related group (DRG). Competitive systems of funding, such as internal markets used in the NHS, have also been used, where hospitals compete for the business of purchasers (insurance companies or GPs) thus providing incentives to reduce costs.

The evidence for each of these methods of payment is mixed.[7] Most evidence on prospective payment is from the USA and the system of DRGs that was used to reimburse hospitals through the federal Medicare programme. Although there is some evidence of cost reductions, it is unclear whether these were achieved by shifting costs to outpatient and long-term care, by reducing quality of care or artificially inflating costs by reclassifying low-cost cases into more expensive cases to maximise the following year's budget.[7]

Evidence on the effects of competition in healthcare markets is also mixed, and depends crucially on the extent of competition within geographical areas. The experience of the UK internal market has, so far, produced little empirical evidence. A review of evidence[8] found that there was some effect on prices, in that lower prices may have been offered to smaller purchasers such as GP fundholders. There was also some evidence that hospital costs were lower, particularly in more competitive areas.

Adverse selection

The third reason why healthcare systems are not dominated by private health insurance is the existence of 'adverse' or risk selection. In a competitive insurance market, insurance companies don't necessarily know what an individual's risk of consuming healthcare is and so a community rated premium (i.e. an average premium across all policy holders) is set. For those individuals who know they are low risk, the premium will be too high and they will choose not to be insured. This leaves the high-risks individuals in the market, but because the community rated premium is too low for this group, it would not cover the expected healthcare costs of such individuals and the insurance company would make losses. This may lead to further rises in premiums, and more people not buying insurance; thus the insurance companies would eventually go out of business.

One response to this is for insurance companies to gather information to try and identify low and high risks. Insurance companies would prefer to insure only the low risks (hence risk selection or 'cream-skimming'), leaving the high risks to face higher premiums and less likely to take out health insurance, resulting in only the healthiest people being covered.

Solutions – universal health insurance coverage

The main concern here is one of equity, as the people most in need of healthcare are not covered by health insurance. A solution to this is to have universal health insurance coverage, where the whole population is covered or to ensure that there are other forms of assistance and subsidies for those who do not have insurance, such as Medicare and Medicaid for the elderly and poor in the USA.

Externalities and public financing of healthcare

The second type of market failure that occurs in healthcare is externalities. These are spillovers from people's activities which effect a third party in either a positive or negative way. Externalities occur when the social costs and benefits of an action do not match the private costs and benefits of the action. For example, if an elderly person receives a hip replacement, their partner will benefit as the patient is less dependent after the operation.

As economic theory assumes that individuals are self-interested, their decisions to purchase healthcare in a market are based on the private costs and benefits of such a purchase. The market does not account for the fact that a decision to purchase healthcare influences the costs or benefits borne by others, as individuals are not willing to pay for these 'extra' benefits or incur the costs (social costs and benefits). It is the costs and benefits that fall on others that are known as externalities (i.e. external effects), which can be either positive or negative. Their existence results in a misallocation of resources such that the market will under or over provide the goods or services (as some costs and benefits have been ignored).

Most externalities in healthcare are positive, in that people benefit from others' use of healthcare services. One of the most obvious forms of externality in healthcare arises because individuals care for the well being of others. This 'caring externality' operates where an individual is altruistic towards others who are ill and are not receiving healthcare. There are also selfish externalities, such as those with immunisation where the treatment of those at risk or who have a contagious disease benefits others, in that they are less likely to contract the disease. These benefits would not be accounted for in a market, thus leading to underprovision of healthcare.

Solutions – public subsidy

The existence of positive externalities suggests that some form of public subsidy or financing of healthcare is appropriate.[7] This may be through taxation or another source of government spending.

Asymmetry of information and the performance and regulation of doctors

The final reason why perfect markets fail in healthcare is that doctors have more information than patients about the effect of healthcare on health status. This creates an agency relationship, where the doctor acts as the patient's agent and can make decisions on their behalf. However, as well as the patient's own objectives (such as improvements in health status), doctors have their own objectives to consider. The imbalance of information puts doctors in an advantageous position that could be used to exploit patients – at the extreme to do harm – but most commonly to recommend treatments that patients would not wish to have, if patients had the same information as doctors. Doctors may do this to increase their own incomes or for other reasons, such as to reduce workload by deciding to refer or prescribe medication. This is known as supplier induced demand (SID), where doctors recommend treatments that patients would not demand if patients had the same information as doctors. As it is not possible to know the treatments patients would have demanded if they had the same information as doctors, it is not possible to test whether supplier induced demand exists. Certainly, doctors do induce demand as agents for patients. However, what is less clear is the extent to which doctors are motivated by their own objectives to the detriment of patients' objectives. Testing whether SID exists is also compounded by the lack of evidence of what does and does not work in healthcare, introducing discretion into doctors' decision making.

Solutions – regulation, payment systems, performance monitoring and doctor–patient communication

Licensure

Licensure ensures that all doctors are qualified and registered and so reduces 'quackery', and can also be used as a basis for self regulation.

Doctor payment systems

Where doctors are paid by FFS, there is a strong incentive to induce demand as there is a direct relationship between doctors' incomes and the volume of services provided. Other forms of payment that sever the link between income and volume of service, such as salary and capitation payment (an annual payment for each patient registered or enrolled) can be introduced, although these have their own incentive effects. For example, it could be argued that capitation payment introduces incentives to minimise effort and encourage referral and prescribing. Several studies have shown that different ways of paying doctors influences their clinical behaviour.[9-12] What is less clear from this literature is whether changes in behaviour represent improvements in efficiency.

Better information is required on the costs and effects of healthcare interventions, coupled with incentives for healthcare providers to use this information. Although such information is now being synthesised using clinical guidelines and regulatory frameworks (such as the National Institute for Clinical Excellence), there is less evidence of its impact on doctors' behaviour, costs and clinical outcomes.[13]

Performance monitoring

Monitoring of performance is part of the clinical governance agenda to improve health service quality, and usually relies on a set of quantitative performance indicators. These are now being used in England and Scotland and are directed at healthcare organisations, such as hospitals. However, it is unclear whether these improve performance for several reasons.[14] First, defining 'performance' using quantitative indicators usually relies on existing data collected for other purposes, and each dimension of performance is usually given equal weight. The relative importance of indicators is usually implicit. Second, the use of targets to improve performance encourages myopia and 'tunnel vision' and diverts resources away from other tasks. Third, external performance monitoring may reduce or 'crowd out' the intrinsic motivation of health providers that motivates them to do a good job because they obtain satisfaction from their work. This area is considered in more detail in Chapter 7.

Addressing doctor–patient information imbalance through improved communication

The above policies deal with symptoms of market failure, rather than their source, which is an imbalance of information in the doctor–patient relationship.[15] Other policies to counter this type of market failure, therefore, include the education of doctors in communication skills, which include providing patients with information and involving them in decision making in consultations. It also involves doctors knowing more about patients' values and preferences, and so continuity of care may be important. Policies to make patients better 'consumers' through the provision of information and involving them more in decision making are also relevant here. Again, there is a great deal of literature in these areas that is beyond the scope of this chapter.[16]

Conclusion

The chapter has provided a brief outline of the main economic issues concerned with healthcare delivery. By considering the main sources of market failure in healthcare, alternative ways of delivering and financing healthcare are suggested. These are wide ranging, and suggest a strong case for government intervention in healthcare delivery to help ensure that:

- the population, particularly low income groups and those in poor health, is covered by publicly provided health insurance with low administrative costs
- incentives are provided to healthcare providers that make them 'cost conscious' through budgets and payment mechanisms
- payment systems, regulation and performance management are designed to encourage healthcare providers to act in their patients' best interests
- patients are given a stronger voice in decisions about their own healthcare.

Several themes emerge from using an economic perspective on healthcare delivery. The first is the central role of patients as consumers of healthcare and the need for healthcare delivery to maximise their objectives. In the perfectly competitive model, consumers are 'sovereign' and this should be replicated when designing systems of healthcare delivery. As well as gathering evidence on which healthcare interventions work, this also involves involving patients in decision making and improving doctor–patient communication.

A second theme is the role of incentives and performance monitoring for healthcare providers. The key here is to ensure that healthcare providers are maximising patients' objectives within available resources, while also attaining their own objectives. If healthcare professionals and managers are subjected to strong external performance monitoring and regulation, they may become demotivated or choose other jobs, introducing problems of recruitment and retention. A balance needs to be struck.

The role of equity in healthcare delivery is the third theme. Depending on society's preferences for equity (which are stronger in Europe than in the USA), this can determine the type and extent of health insurance coverage for a population, and also how healthcare resources are distributed across the population.

Finally, there continues to be a lack of empirical evidence on alternative methods of healthcare delivery and the factors that influence it. As with changes in clinical practice, changes in healthcare delivery or financing should be evaluated in terms of their effects on costs and on benefits to patients, as well as examining their effects on the behaviour of healthcare providers.

Acknowledgements

The Health Economics Research Unit is funded by the Chief Scientist's Office of the Scottish Executive Health Department (SEHD). Thanks to Shelley Farrar, John Cairns and David Kernick for comments on an earlier draft. The views in this paper are those of the author and not the SEHD.

References

1   Arrow KJ (1963) The welfare economics of medical care. *Am Economic Rev.* **53**: 941–73.
2   Zweifel P and Manning W (2000) Moral hazard and consumer incentives in healthcare. In: AJ Culyer and JP Newhouse (eds) *Handbook of Health Economics.* Volume 1A. Elsevier, Amsterdam.
3   Croxson B, Propper C and Perkins A (2001) Do doctors respond to financial incentives? UK family doctors and the GP fundholder scheme. *J Public Economics.* **79**: 375–98.
4   LeGrand J, Mays N and Mulligan J (1998) *Learning from the NHS Internal Market: a review of the evidence.* King's Fund Publishing, London.
5   Hillman AL, Pauly MV and Kernstein JJ (1989) How do financial incentives affect physicians' clinical decisions and the financial performance of health maintenance organisations? *NEJM.* **321**: 86–92.
6   Glied S (2000) Managed care. In: AJ Culyer and JP Newhouse (eds) *Handbook of Health Economics.* Volume 1A. Elsevier, Amsterdam.
7   Donaldson C and Gerard K (1992) *Economics of Healthcare Financing: the visible hand.* Macmillan, London.
8   Propper C and Sodelund N (1998) Competition in the NHS internal market: an overview of its effects on hospital prices and costs. *Health Economics.* **7**: 187–97.
9   Gosden T, Gosden T, Forland F *et al.* (2000) Capitation, salary, fee-for-service and mixed systems of payment: effects on the behaviour of primary care physicians (Systematic review). Cochrane Effective Practice and Organisation of Care Group, Cochrane Database of Systematic Reviews. Issue 3.
10 Kransik A, Groenewegen PP, Pedersen PA *et al.* (1990) Changing remuneration systems: effects on activity in general practice. *BMJ.* **360**: 1698–701.
11 Scott A and Hall J (1995) Evaluating the effects of GP remuneration: problems and prospects. *Health Policy.* **31**: 183–95.
12 Guiffrida A and Gravelle H (2001) Inducing or restraining demand: the market for night visits in primary care. *J Health Economics.* **20**: 755–80.

13 Grimshaw JM, Shirran L, Thomas RE, Mowatt G, Fraser C and Bero L (In press) Changing provider behaviour: an overview of systematic reviews of interventions. *Med Care*.

14 Goddard M, Mannion R and Smith P (2000) Enhancing performance in healthcare: a theoretical perspective on agency and the role of information. *Health Economics*. **9**: 95-107.

15 Scott A (2001) Health economics and patient choice. In: A Edwards and G Elwyn (eds) *Evidence-Based Patient Choice*. Oxford University Press, Oxford.

16 Bekker H, Thornton JG, Airey CM *et al.* (1999) Informed decision making: an annotated bibliography and systematic review. *Health Technol Assess*. **3(1)**.

CHAPTER 3

Using health economics to facilitate decision making: the basics of economic evaluation

David Kernick and Ruth McDonald

The area of health economics that will be of most relevance to practitioners, commissioners and managers and that forms the core of this book is economic evaluation. Economic evaluation is the comparison of resource implications and benefits of alternative ways of delivering healthcare. This chapter introduces some basic concepts underpinning this analytical framework which seeks to facilitate decision making against a background of scarce resources.

Key points

- Economic evaluation can facilitate decisions in a way that is both transparent and fair. It offers a framework in which a comparative analysis of alternative courses of action in terms of their costs and consequences can be studied.
- Four key concepts underpin economic evaluation – scarcity and sacrifice, efficiency, opportunity cost, and utility.
- It is important to be clear about the perspective or viewpoint of an economic analysis. This will determine which costs and benefits are relevant.
- Health economists stress the importance of measuring a wide range of costs. Some of these may be difficult to quantify in monetary terms.
- The way in which benefits are measured characterises the type of economic evaluation.

- As the relationship between costs and benefits is rarely expressed by a simple proportional relationship, it is important to identify how increments in benefit change with increments in cost.

Chapter sections
- **Introduction**
- **Four key health economic concepts**
- **The concept of economic evaluation**
- **Conclusion**

Introduction

Commissioners and providers of healthcare are being asked to make judgements about the relative merits of different interventions that lead to decisions about resource allocation. Health economics is a subdiscipline of economics, which focuses on the allocation of healthcare resources in a world where demands exceed resources.

The growing pressures on health budgets make it increasingly important for decisions to be made in a manner that is both fair and transparent. Economic evaluation offers a framework in which a comparative analysis of alternative courses of action, in terms of both their costs and consequences and the values attached to them, can be undertaken to facilitate the inevitable difficult choices (Figure 3.1).

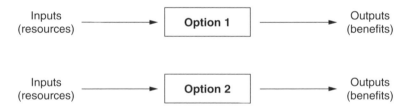

Figure 3.1:   An economic analysis relates inputs (resources) to outputs (benefits and the values attached to them) of alternative interventions to facilitate decision making when resources are scarce.

Although health economists are interested in a number of areas as outlined in Chapter 1, economic analysis forms a major part of their work. It is the area of health economics that will be of most relevance to practitioners, commissioners and managers and forms the core of this book. Before we can understand economic evaluation, four key concepts must be described that underpin health economic theory.

Four key health economic concepts

Scarcity and sacrifice

Because resources are scarce, choices have to be made about how to consume these resources. Sacrifice is inevitable – not everyone can receive the healthcare that will do them some good.

Efficiency

The concept of efficiency is central to health economics. In general, efficiency refers to getting the most out of limited resources, either by achieving a given output from the minimum possible input or producing the maximum possible from a fixed resource. Efficiency advocates the adoption of two basic principles: to ensure that sacrifices entailed are kept to a minimum and that no activity is pursued unless the benefits gained outweigh the benefits foregone.

Opportunity cost

The notion of 'opportunity cost' is central to economic analysis and reflects the fact that resources are scarce and that choices have to be made about the best ways of allocating them. When deciding to spend resources on a new treatment, those resources cannot now be used for other healthcare programmes or treatments. The opportunity cost of the new treatment is the value of the next best alternative use of those resources. Unlike accountancy there is more to costs than the spending of money. Cost is viewed as sacrifice rather than financial expenditure.

For example, consider the cost of a GP increasing consultation time by an extra hour. The GP may work the same number of hours but reduce services provided in other areas so the opportunity cost is the value of the services displaced. Alternatively, the working week may be extended so the opportunity cost is that of the GP's leisure time. In practice, the most appropriate estimate of the cost will depend on the context of the evaluation and the perspective of the exercise. Note that health economists seek to value elements such as leisure time which do not normally attract a financial cost.

Utility

Utility is the value an individual places on a health state. Health economists seek to measure utility from healthcare interventions in order to compare their relative value for money. Generally, two main methods for assessing utility are used.

- People with a particular health state are asked to value that state based on their own preference.
- People who do not have this health state are asked to place a value on it. This could be members of the public based on a description of the health state, or clinicians who have some experience of treating patients with this health state.

Utilities are assigned values of between 1 (best possible health) and 0 (death).

The concept of economic evaluation

An economic evaluation relates inputs (resources and the values attached to them) to outputs (benefits and the values attached to them) of alternative interventions to facilitate decision making when resources are scarce. Economic evaluations always consider outcomes as well as costs, although they differ with regard to the valuation of outcomes. Here we give a basic description of economic evaluation, which is considered more fully in Section 3.

Economic evaluation seeks to organise and clarify information so as to facilitate decision making. It can help decision makers to choose between healthcare interventions with the aim of maximising health benefit. For example, should a primary care trust increase spending on coronary artery bypass grafts or hip replacements? Alternatively, it can examine different ways to meet a particular objective at least cost. For example, how should heart failure be treated? Should doctors or nurses deliver asthma care?

The perspective of an analysis

Economic evaluations are undertaken from a particular viewpoint. This will determine which costs and benefits to quantify.[1] The viewpoint could be a societal, NHS, primary care group, GP practice or patient perspective. Most economic studies adopt an NHS perspective but in general, health economists advocate a societal viewpoint which takes into account all relevant costs and benefits. For example, in addition to NHS expenditure, costs falling on social services, to individuals and their families, to the public purse generally and costs to the economy, in terms of lost productivity, would be included. NHS viewpoints may not always concur with those of other interested parties such as the primary care trust or GP practice. When considering the results of an economic evaluation, it is important to ascertain the perspective from which it has been undertaken and to ensure that all relevant costs and consequences have been included from the perspective of the decision maker.

The importance of marginal analysis

Most decisions in healthcare are concerned with the expansion or contraction of services (i.e. changes at the margin). As the relationship between costs and

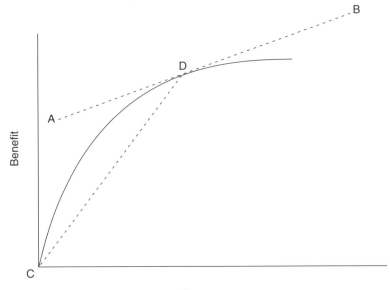

Figure 3.2: Benefits do not continue to increase in a simple proportional relationship as more resources are invested in any healthcare intervention. It is important to relate increments in resources invested to the incremental increase in benefits. The gradient of A–B represents the marginal cost/benefit ratio, which is quite different from the gradient C–D, the average cost/benefit ratio.

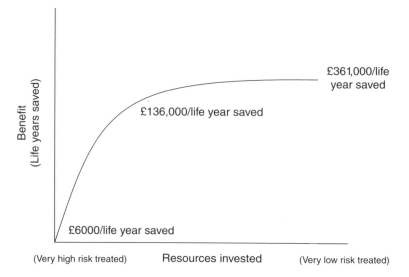

Figure 3.3:   The costs and benefits in terms of life years saved from statin treatment. Costs/life year saved are shown for very high risk, low risk and very low risk patients.[3]

benefits can rarely be expressed by a straight line, health economists stress the importance of analysing changes in terms of their marginal effects.[2] A marginal analysis identifies how increments in benefit change with increments in cost (Figure 3.2). Note that at any point of resource investment, the marginal cost per unit of benefit differs from the average cost per unit of benefit.

Figure 3.3 demonstrates this principle and shows how the benefits of using statin drugs in terms of cost/year of life saved change as more resources are directed to treating patients at lower risk. For low-risk patients £361,000 will have to be spent to save a year of life compared with only £6000 for very high risk groups.

Measuring benefits in an economic evaluation

Although patients can receive satisfaction from non-health related benefits, such as reassurance, choice, information and availability of medical services, in practice economic evaluation has focused on more tangible or measurable health related outcomes. There are four main methods of economic evaluation that are characterised by the benefits that are measured as shown in Table 3.1. These are considered in more depth in Section 3.

Table 3.1: The four types of formal economic evaluation

Form of evaluation	Measurement and valuation of outcomes
Cost minimisation analysis	Outcomes are assumed to be equivalent. Focus of measurement is on costs. Not often relevant as outcomes are rarely equivalent
Cost effectiveness analysis	Natural units (e.g. life years gained, deaths prevented). This approach forms the bulk of published studies and will be of most relevance to practitioners
Cost utility analysis	Health state values based on individual preferences (e.g. quality adjusted life years gained). An approach which is gaining in importance due to the need to decide between different interventions at a national level and the importance placed on quality of life. Many methodological problems remain
Cost benefit analysis	All outcomes valued in monetary units (e.g. valuation of amount willing to pay to prevent a death). Rarely used due to methodological problems in valuing all outcomes in monetary terms

Cost minimisation analysis

In cost minimisation analysis, the consequences of two or more interventions being compared are equivalent. The analysis therefore focuses on costs alone, although the evidence of equivalent outcomes should be established prior to consideration of costs.

Cost effectiveness analysis

Cost effectiveness analysis[4] is used to compare drugs or programmes which have a common health outcome (e.g. reduction in blood pressure, life years saved). Results are usually presented in the form of a ratio (e.g. costs per life year gained).

If two treatments A and B are compared and costs are lower for A and outcomes better, then treatment A is said to dominate. If, as is more commonly the case with a new drug, costs are higher for one treatment, but benefits are higher too, it is necessary to calculate how much extra benefit is obtained for the extra cost. A decision then needs to be made as to whether this addition in benefit is worth paying for.

Often, intermediate or surrogate outcomes such as cases detected and reduction in cholesterol are measured, and it is important to ensure that these intermediate measures have clinical meaning in terms of long-term outcome for patients.

Cost utility analysis

Often, interventions impact both on quality and quantity of life. Where this is the case, cost utility analysis[5] can be used to assess costs and benefits of interventions. The most frequently used measure is the quality adjusted life year (QALY). Benefits are measured based on impact on length and quality of life to produce an overall index of health gain. QALYs reflect people's preferences for different health states, but their use remains contested in a number of areas.

Cost benefit analysis

In a cost benefit analysis,[6] attempts are made to value all the costs and consequences of an intervention in monetary terms. The data requirements for this approach are large, and methodological issues around the valuation of non-monetary benefits such as lives saved make this method problematic.

Cost consequences analysis

In some cases, studies consider multiple outcomes rather than condense benefits into a single measure.[7] Costs and outcomes are presented in a disaggregated form, which avoids the need to represent results as a single index. Although this approach is not a formal method of economic analysis and as such is not shown in Table 3.1, it is one that may be more attractive to decision makers who can apply their own weight to the various outcomes.

Measuring costs in an economic evaluation

An accurate assessment of costs will be an important part of any economic evaluation. How costs are derived and combined will depend on the assumptions that have been made in their derivation. It is important to be clear about the assumptions that have been made and why, in order to maintain consistency across comparative studies and prevent inappropriate conclusions being drawn.[8] Costing principles and concepts are considered in more depth in Section 3. Table 3.2 shows some cost definitions used in health economics.

Direct costs are those costs associated directly with a healthcare intervention (e.g. physician salaries, patient transport costs). However, health economists recognise the importance of valuing a broad range of cost inputs rather than only those items for which a market price is readily available or which impact on the NHS budget. For example, indirect costs incurred by patients in terms of loss of employment or leisure time may be an important contribution, but the calculation of such costs is problematical. Intangible costs such as the

Table 3.2:   Cost definitions used in health economics

Direct costs	Costs associated directly with a healthcare intervention (e.g. GP salaries, drug costs)
Indirect costs	Costs associated with reduced productivity due to illness, disability or death
Intangible costs	The cost of pain and suffering occurring as a result of illness or treatment
Marginal cost	The extra cost of one extra unit of service provided

cost of pain or suffering are even more difficult to quantify in monetary terms. The costs to be included in any study will depend on the study perspective. Studies which take a societal perspective usually include both direct and indirect costs.

Conclusion

By providing an explicit framework for considering alternatives, economic evaluation can help decision makers move beyond gut feeling towards a more systematic approach to decision making by framing the questions that are asked. However, this approach has yet to make a significant impact on decision making, particularly at grassroots level. Economic evaluation is considered in more detail in Section 3 and the problems of applying it in practice in Section 4.

References

1 Byford S and Raftery J (1998) Perspectives in economic evaluation. *BMJ.* **316:** 152–9.
2 Torgerson DJ and Spencer A (1996) Marginal costs and benefits. *BMJ.* **312:** 35–6.
3 Pharoah P and Hollingworth W (1996) Cost effectiveness of lowering cholesterol concentration with statins in patients with and without existing coronary heart disease. *BMJ.* **312:** 1443–8.
4 Robinson R (1993) Cost effective analysis. *BMJ.* **307:** 793–5.
5 Robinson R (1993) Cost utility analysis. *BMJ.* **307:** 859–62.
6 Robinson R (1993) Cost benefit analysis. *BMJ.* **307:** 924–6.
7 Mauskopf J, Paul J, Grant D *et al.* (1998) The role of cost consequence analysis in healthcare decision making. *Pharmacoeconomics.* **13(3):** 277–88.
8 Kernick D (2000) Costing principles in primary care. *Family Practice.* **17:** 66–70.

Section 2

Aspects of health economics

In this section, we look at a number of areas where health economists contribute to policy making and healthcare organisation. John Appleby opens by describing how we allocate budgets at different levels of the health service and how health economists contribute to this process. In private healthcare markets, healthcare spending is simply the sum of the decisions of purchasers. Inevitably, in a public system based on need and not the ability to pay, resource allocation decisions are not going to be easy.

One way of measuring the impact of a disease area on society is to measure its economic burden. In Chapter 5, I review cost of illness studies. Although popular with pharmaceutical companies who use them to emphasise the importance of a disease area, health economists tend to treat them with a degree of caution. It is argued that what is important is not the cost of an illness but how that burden can be improved by investing limited resources in it.

The NHS Plan proposes a radical redesign of the whole system of healthcare, and there have been calls from successive governments for closer integration between health and social care sectors. However, political, professional and cultural obstacles have hindered genuine progress in this area. In Chapter 6, Martin Knapp and Ann Netten consider the challenges of integrating health and social care from the health economists' perspective. They do not underestimate the problems ahead.

Another central tenet of the government's attempt to modernise the NHS has been the development of the clinical governance agenda – a framework to improve quality and accountability of clinical care. In Chapter 7, Russell Mannion and Huw Davies offer some economic insights using the principal–agent framework and uncover some of the key tensions that lie at the heart of clinical governance policies.

One of the biggest changes in the NHS since its inception has been the split between purchasers and providers of healthcare. In Chapter 8, Ray Robinson explores the costs of buying and selling services and demonstrates that although transaction costs have an important influence on the way in which the healthcare system is structured, in practice they are often difficult to measure.

CHAPTER 4

How much should we spend on healthcare and how should we distribute it?

John Appleby

One of the fundamental principles of the NHS is that care should be based on need and not ability to pay. In private healthcare markets, healthcare spending is simply the sum of the decisions of purchasers. In a public system, however, decisions must be made about total spending levels and how to allocate resources at all levels. This chapter reviews how these decisions are made across the NHS and the input of health economics into them.

Key points
- In a private healthcare market, no decisions are taken by anyone as to the total spending in the market.
- A publicly funded system raises difficult issues about the total level of spending, and how resources should be distributed – ranging from NHS budget setting to resource decisions at the treatment level.
- In theory, health economists would suggest that total NHS spending should be set at the point where one more pound spent would produce additional health valued at just under one pound.
- In practice, how much is spent on healthcare is a combination of historical precedent, public opinion, affordability and international comparison.
- Health economists have developed formulae for allocating the NHS budget across the country to reflect different need for healthcare in different areas.

- Health economists are exerting an increasing impact on decisions in areas that have previously been the prerogative of clinicians.

Chapter sections
- Introduction
- Setting the NHS budget – distribution at the macro level
- Sharing out the NHS budget – distribution at the meso level
- Spending the NHS budget – distribution at the micro level
- Conclusion

Introduction

Deciding how much to spend on the NHS in the UK has been a (literally and metaphorically) taxing question for all governments since 1948.[1-3] For a public service funded mainly from general taxation, setting a budget for the NHS every year raises difficult political, macroeconomic, technical and, indeed, ethical issues. Having reached a decision on the global NHS budget, the subsidiary question of how it is to be distributed then raises further difficult issues concerning rationing/priority setting and additional ethical issues such as fairness and equity. The task of deciding the distribution (or allocation) of society's scarce resources covers not only the determination of the global healthcare budget, but reoccurs at various stages within the healthcare system all the way down to decisions taken by individual clinicians faced with individual patients (Figure 4.1). Other chapters deal in more detail with issues of rationing at these lower levels in the system. However, following a review of ways to determine the global NHS budget, distribution at the meso level (dividing up the global budget within the system) is covered, followed by an overview of rationing decisions at the sharp end of the NHS.

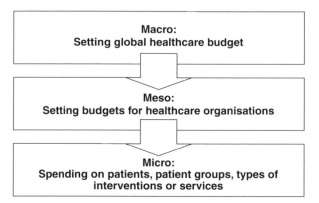

Figure 4.1:   Resource allocation decisions in healthcare.

Before considering how global budgets have been determined and the approaches taken to distribution and priority setting, it is helpful to contrast the tasks facing the NHS in these areas with the way a private market in healthcare would deal with them. The main point to note about a private healthcare market is that no decision is taken by anyone as to the total spending in the market! Total spending is simply an outcome of all the many decisions made by purchasers and providers in the market. Purchasers will make their own decisions about how much healthcare to buy based partly on their perceived needs for care and constrained by their personal incomes and their desires to spend their incomes on other, non-healthcare, goods and services. How much is spent in total in the market is of little concern to individual purchasers.

For the NHS (and like many similar public healthcare systems) a key driver in private markets, the link between an individual's ability to pay and their consumption of healthcare has been deliberately broken; most agree that access to healthcare should be based on need, not ability to pay. However, having eliminated this link, the NHS is then faced with a top-down decision about its total budget. By contrast with a private market, total spending becomes a key concern for patients and the public. Governments and their 'agents' (primary care groups, GPs etc.) have to take charge of functions (budget setting, distribution etc.) which a private market would otherwise perform automatically in a bottom-up way.

If decisions about healthcare spending are not made by individuals, how do governments approach making decisions on spending and distribution on our behalf, and is there a 'right' level of spending? The rest of this chapter describes economic and other approaches to these issues. It will become clear that while economic ideas and techniques have a part to play, there is no straightforward technical solution to determine spending levels – for the NHS it is ultimately a political decision.

Setting the NHS budget – distribution at the macro level

An economist's approach to setting the NHS budget

Paul Samuelson's compact definition of the fundamentals of economics (Box 4.1) contains a key concept which suggests how an economist would tackle the budget setting question for the NHS – resources are scarce.[4]

Box 4.1:   A definition of economics[4]

[Economics is] the study of how people and society end up choosing, with or without the use of money, to employ scarce productive resources that could have alternative uses, to produce various commodities and distribute them for consumption, now or in the future, among various people and groups in society. It analyses the costs and benefits of improving patterns of resource allocation.

From an economic point of view, the government has to make a choice as to how to employ its tax and other revenues. These resources are scarce in the economic sense that there will always be more calls on its total budget than money available. Of course, governments often try and circumvent this fundamental problem by borrowing, but this is not a sustainable solution to the scarcity problem. If the choice is between spending on healthcare, education, roads, defence and so on, as well as leaving taxpayers with the choice to spend their own disposable incomes as they wish, then how, in crude terms, is the government to decide how to carve up the cake?

Hospitals and schools all cost money, but the reason for spending on these is that they produce benefits – health, education and so on. Furthermore, higher spending tends to produce greater benefits. The exact relationship between costs (spending) and benefits is not straightforward, however, and certainly not linear. The economist's equivalent of the physicist's universal law is that of diminishing returns. Simply put, it states that as the inputs (money) to a process (healthcare) are increased there comes a point when the value of the outputs (healthiness, say), while still increasing, do so at a decreasing rate, and eventually may well start to decrease in absolute terms (equivalent to making a patient more unwell by overtreating).

If the choice was simplified to one where the only spending option was the NHS, then healthcare spending should be set at a level where just one more pound spent would produce a health outcome worth just less than a pound. The economist's advice would be to stop spending when marginal costs equalled marginal benefits (at the point where the curve showing marginal returns for different levels of spending starts to turn in Figure 4.2).

For governments the choice is more complicated, and involves reaching a decision about spending not only on the NHS but education, defence and so on. In this case, the first call on the government's finite resources should be for those areas which produce the greatest benefits (which might or might not be the NHS). Investment would increase up to the point where greater benefits can be obtained by spending in another area (education, say), and so on until revenues run out.

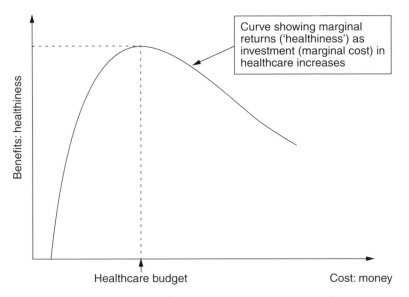

Figure 4.2: Decreasing returns to healthcare investment.

Clearly, this latter process requires the outcomes (benefits) of all government spending to be measured in common units (such as money). While economists have developed ways of valuing the apparently impossible-to-value (the Department of Transport regularly use a value for a statistical human life in its cost benefit analyses of transport schemes, for example), the information requirements alone of the economist's approach to budget setting is prohibitive.

Moreover, the essential notion or bottom line underlying the economist's decision rule about spending is efficiency – maximising outcome for a given level of input. Obtaining the biggest 'bang per buck', however, is not always the overriding criterion for the NHS (or indeed most healthcare systems). Other objectives, such as equity, may well be deemed as or more important than efficiency. However, the economist's approach to budget setting does not necessarily preclude the use of criteria other than efficiency. The key consideration is clarity about what each healthcare pound is meant to buy. So, for example, in Figure 4.2, 'healthiness' could be defined in terms of quality adjusted life years (QALYs), and using the efficiency criterion alone would suggest that the global healthcare budget should be set at the point at which spending one more pound buys less QALYs than the previous pound. The efficiency criterion, however, ignores the distribution of QALYs across a population. Theoretically at least, it is possible to adjust QALYs to reflect some notion of equity so that each healthcare pound not only buys QALYs, but a certain distribution of QALYs across a population which reflects society's desire for fairness.

As already mentioned, a central problem with the economist's approach is the enormous amount of information needed. Nonetheless, the ideas which underpin this method can be helpful not only at a national level* but also locally. NHS commissioning organisations face similar resource allocation decisions, and have to decide, within a fixed budget, how much to spend on different types of care for different population groups. One practical application of the economist's approach is programme budgeting and marginal analysis (*see* Chapter 18).

Other approaches

Incrementalism

Historically, the Department of Health has tended to set spending levels for the NHS in an incremental way, using past budgets as a baseline and then adding further amounts to reflect demand pressures on the system – such as changes in the demographic structure of the population, the costs of new healthcare technologies, overall changes in the need for healthcare services and so on.[5] Although having the advantage of practicality, it is fairly crude and relies on the circular logic that last year's budget was set at the 'correct' level and that all that is required is to adjust it at the margins. As a necessity, this method also has to make assumptions about the impact demand pressures will have on the NHS budget. For example, it is not clear that new medical technologies necessarily add to total NHS cost. While often costing more than existing interventions at a patient level, overall, new technologies may lead to lower total costs.

Public opinion

An alternative method to determining spending levels is to ascertain what the public would like to spend on healthcare. Opinion polls have for many years consistently revealed that the public agree that more should be spent on the NHS.[6,7] However, it is difficult to know how such polls should be interpreted or, indeed, what credence to attach to the results of what is essentially a hypothetical question. As such polls do not require the public to actually support their views with real money, respondents will inevitably undervalue the opportunity costs of their desire to spend more on the NHS – leading to a bias in the answers they give. Unlike a market, where decisions to spend more on healthcare naturally means a concomitant decision to spend less on other things (the opportunity cost being the value of the benefits foregone as a result of such a decision), expressing an opinion is costless!

---

*For example, in formulating its guidance to the NHS, the National Institute for Clinical Excellence (NICE) draws heavily on economic evaluation techniques to reach decisions about cost effectiveness.

Nevertheless, in a democratic system, opinion polls – in the form of general elections – could be said to influence healthcare spending, with voting partly determined by manifesto pledges on healthcare spending. Although for much of the 1980s and 1990s, there was a contradictory tendency for the electorate to express an opinion that more should be spent on healthcare while voting for a party which had a record of parsimony in this area, recent general election results suggest a convergence.

Affordability

The notion of opportunity cost noted above combined with the incrementalist approach could be used at a national level in order to determine annual changes in healthcare spending. Some commentators have suggested that changes in NHS spending should be linked to changes in the wealth of the country (as measured by, for example, gross domestic product (GDP)).[8] In a sense, this treats the economy as if it were like the budget of a household and brings home the impact of spending more on healthcare nationally – that is, spending less on other things. Practically however, there are a number of problems with this approach. First, it requires some initial decision as to the share of national wealth to be devoted to healthcare. Second, it also requires decisions about the stability of this share – should it increase sometimes or should it remain as a fixed percentage (in which case, in times of recession, less will be spent on healthcare – just when we might well need to spend more)? Third, it requires somebody to take these decisions.

International comparisons

A fourth approach to the problem combines the affordability method noted above with some objective evidence concerning one of the problems with this approach – the decision about the appropriate share of the national budget that should be devoted to healthcare.

Figure 4.3 shows that there is a significant association between the per capita wealth of a country and its per capita healthcare spending. The association is not perfect, of course, but is statistically strong and suggests that as a country's wealth increases so it tends to devote a higher proportion of that wealth to healthcare.

This association can be used to set spending levels. For the UK – slightly below the line – this would mean increasing spending to the level we might expect given the UK's GDP. For some other countries, such as Germany, this approach would suggest reducing spending. While this approach contains some underlying economic rationale – the notion of opportunity cost, for example – the reliance on comparisons with other countries is difficult to justify.[9]

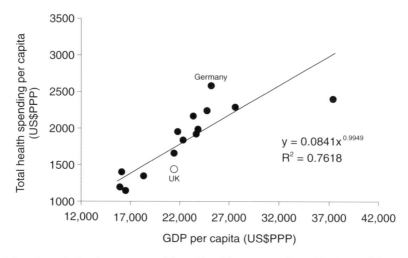

Figure 4.3:   Association between wealth and healthcare spending. (OECD Health Data 2000, projections by the author.)

Sharing out the NHS budget – distribution at the meso level

Following ministerial concern about the uneven distribution of services across the country, the approach taken to distributing the global NHS budget took a leap forward in the mid 1970s with the use of needs-based formula based on work by the Resource Allocation Working Party (RAWP). Its guiding criterion for determining budgets for administrative healthcare organisations was equity – interpreted (for practical reasons) by the working party as equity of access to healthcare, and operationalised through the use of mortality and demographic data to determine shares of the total healthcare budget.

RAWP has undergone various revisions, and now operates as a weighted capitation system, with refined census-derived variables serving to reflect the differential need for healthcare in different (geographical) areas. Part of these changes also attempted to address the fact that supply and demand in healthcare are not, as traditionally assumed by economists, independent of each other.[10] Supply can influence demand; indeed, supply can induce demand.

Recent government proposals to revise the underlying criterion for the weighted capitation system – to include an objective of distributing financial resources to reduce avoidable health inequalities[11] – raise some difficult practical issues as well as the extent to which health (as opposed to access to healthcare) can be influenced by the NHS resource allocation system.[12] Over the last few years, significant chunks of the total NHS budget have begun to bypass the weighted capitation system, to be directed through the health modernisation fund, at specific initiatives and services deemed priorities by government.[13]

Moves to primary care trusts (PCTs) and the abolition of health authorities will not change the essentials of the method of sharing out the cake in the NHS (although with the demise of health authorities, PCTs will receive their cash limited budgets direct from the Department of Health on the basis of the national weighted capitation formula).

Spending the NHS budget – distribution at the micro level

Setting the national NHS budget (choosing between healthcare and non-healthcare spending) and then deciding how to share out the NHS budget geographically (and latterly, through the modernisation fund on the basis of disease-specific services, cancer, heart disease etc.) leads inexorably to the most difficult distributional question – who to treat? It is at this micro level that health economics has generated the most controversy.

Within the section above on deciding the national allocation to healthcare, a common unit of currency for measuring benefits – QALYs – was noted as one way to assess the returns to investment in healthcare, and by extension, an even more common currency – money – was suggested as a unit to assess invest-ment or spending levels across all government activity. The same approach (i.e. finding a common unit of outcome or benefit) could also, at least in theory, be used at the micro level of distribution, with the spending decision rule again based on the efficiency criterion – interventions or patients able to 'generate' the least costly QALYs being the first to attract spending. Subsequent interven-tions or patients would then attract funds up to the point where the total budget was exhausted. Beyond this level of spending there will of course exist people who are ill and for whom there exist effective treatments, but the combined macro, meso and micro budget setting decisions have meant that they will not be treated.

However, it is not just opponents of this approach that can recognise the ethi-cal dilemmas it raises. Economists too are aware that following such a decision rule would lead to outcomes many would find objectionable. For example, using QALYs as a health status measure[†] naturally means that the young will have, on average, a greater capacity to generate QALYs than the elderly. If cost per

---

† Not an unreasonable attempt at capturing two key dimensions of health – length and qual-ity of life.

QALY were used as the basis for rationing scarce healthcare resources, the elderly, many have argued (for example, Grimley Evans (1997)[14]), would therefore be discriminated against purely on the basis of their age.

Such arguments miss the point, however. As also noted earlier, other decision criteria – such as equity – are of course necessary in reaching desirable decisions (and outcomes) in healthcare. The value judgement is, therefore, determining the criteria that should be adopted (or, more precisely, determining the balance that should be reached between competing criteria). In the case of the age discrimination argument (which arises implicitly from the degree to which individuals have the capacity to benefit from healthcare and which is, therefore, an indirect discrimination), an economic approach to the issue would not be prescriptive, but would point out that pursuing an equality objective (all have access to care irrespective of their capacity to benefit, for example) is only achievable at great (opportunity) cost.

In practice, treatment decisions at the level of individual patients have been and largely remain the prerogative of clinicians. The basis for treatment decisions is, in general, based on clinical considerations. However, clinical decisions are clearly taken within the wider context of resource constraints (for a hospital, the NHS as a whole) and as such rationing choices have to be made (hence, for example, the existence of waiting lists). Moreover, criteria such as capacity to benefit, equity and indeed, financial factors are not ignored by clinicians. Whether some form of economic evaluation is carried out implicitly or explicitly, it is inevitable that it is done. The key argument, therefore, is the extent to which economic evaluation is overt. Economists would argue that, on grounds of fairness and consistency in the treatment of patients, rationing decisions which have traditionally been hidden should be more transparent.[†]

This is not an easy task, of course, and requires all decision makers in the NHS (clinicians, commissioning organisations, NICE etc.) to not only be clear about their objectives, but to achieve consistency in their decision criteria.

Conclusion

While economics can provide a way of thinking about how to determine total healthcare budgets, there are – as economists would be the first to recognise – practical problems with their approach. Left to our own devices and with a market for healthcare, an equilibrium would be reached which would provide a figure (albeit relatively meaningless in terms of the market) for total spending on healthcare. However, such an amount cannot be considered the 'right'

---

† Unexplained variations in rates of hospitalisation, referrals, prescribing and many other clinical activities perhaps reinforce the need for greater transparency of clinical decision making.

amount to spend. Indeed, for a public healthcare system which has deliberately broken the link between personal income and personal consumption of care, this figure would certainly be the wrong amount, and, more importantly, be derived from a distribution of consumption significantly based on the distribution of consumers' incomes.

Ultimately, how much should be spent on the NHS is primarily a subjective question of political and public choice based on agreed objectives for the service and desired outcomes, but constrained by competing calls on society's finite resources. Health economics has a role to play in suggesting frameworks within which to make the decision, generating the appropriate technical information and also in assessing the consequences of proposed courses of action.

How the healthcare budget is then distributed – across geographical areas and individuals in need of care – raises further difficult technical and ethical questions. Again, a key role for economics is to suggest frameworks for thinking through and, importantly separating out these ethical and technical issues. Ultimately, economics and economic evaluation is not just something that economists do – anyone taking a decision involving the use of resources for which there are competing claims is 'doing economics'.

References

1   Appleby J (1992) *Financing Health Care in the 1990s*. Open University Press, Buckingham.
2   Dixon J, Harrison A and New B (1997) Is the NHS underfunded? *BMJ*. **314:** 58–61.
3   Appleby J and Boyle S (2000) Blair's billions: where will he find the money for the NHS? *BMJ*. **320:** 865–7.
4   Samuelson PA (1980) *Economics* (11e). McGraw-Hill, London.
5   Smee CH (1996) Setting regional allocations and national budgets in the UK. In: FW Schwartz, H Glennerster and RB Saltman (eds) *Fixing Health Budgets: experience from Europe and North America*. Wiley, Chichester.
6   Judge K and Soloman M (1993) Public opinion and the National Health Service: patterns and perspectives in consumer satisfaction. *J Social Policy*. **22(3):** 299–327.
7   Mulligan J-A (2001) The battle for public opinion. In: J Appleby and A Harrison (eds) *Health Care UK Autumn 2001*. King's Fund, London.
8   O'Higgins M (1987) *Health Spending: a way of sustainable growth*. Institute of Health Services Management/Royal College of Nursing/BMA, London.
9   Appleby J and Boyle S (2001) NHS spending: the wrong target (again)? In: J Appleby and A Harrison (eds) *Health Care UK Spring 2001*. King's Fund, London.
10 Carr-Hill RA, Sheldon TA, Smith P, Martin S, Peacock S and Hardman G (1994) Allocating resources to health authorities: development of methods for small area analysis of use of inpatient services. *BMJ*. **309:** 1046–9.
11 Department of Health (2001) website: www.doh.goc.uk/allocations/review (viewed 8/11/01).

12 Smith P, Shaw R and Hauck K (2000) *Reducing Avoidable Inequalities in Health: a new criterion for setting healthcare capitations.* Centre for Health Economics, University of York, York.

13 Appleby J (1999) Datascan: the modernisation fund. In: J Appleby and A Harrison (eds) *Health Care UK 1999/2000 Edition.* King's Fund, London.

14 Grimley Evans J (1997) Rationing health care by age: rejoinder to Alan Williams. In: B New (ed.) *Rationing: talk and action in health care.* King's Fund/BMJ, London.

CHAPTER 5

Measuring the economic burden of illness

David Kernick

Cost of illness studies aim to quantify the burden of disease by expressing it in monetary terms. Although these studies are popular with the pharmaceutical industry who use them to highlight the importance of a particular disease area, many health economists remain unconvinced of their value. The economic cost of an illness can help to determine research priorities, but should not be used to allocate resources unless it can be demonstrated that cost effective interventions can lower the economic burden.

Key points
- Cost of illness studies aim to quantify the burden of a disease by expressing it in monetary terms.
- Direct costs form the cornerstone of cost of illness studies and reflect the costs borne by the healthcare system such as drugs and hospital admissions. Indirect costs arising from productivity losses and intangible costs, such as the costs allocated to pain and suffering, are less easy to measure.
- Cost of illness studies should not be used to allocate treatment resources unless there is good evidence to suggest that cost effective interventions are available that will reduce this burden.

Chapter sections
- What is a cost of illness study?
- What types of cost of illness studies are there?
- What do cost of illness studies measure?
- Can cost of illness studies help decision makers?
- Other economic approaches to burden of illness
- Conclusion

What is a cost of illness study?

Cost of illness or economic burden of illness studies offer an alternative perspective on the importance of diseases compared with other epidemiological indicators such as morbidity and mortality. Many illnesses create a burden for patients, their families and society, and cost of illness studies aim to quantify this burden by measuring all the costs of a particular disease in monetary terms.[1,2]

The exercise is a three-stage process:

- define the disease
- itemise the resource implications
- value and sum these elements.

Unlike an economic evaluation that values the inputs of a healthcare intervention, cost of illness studies value the consequences of a disease. However, the methodology of costing is similar in both exercises.

What types of cost of illness studies are there?

Cost of illness studies can be undertaken according to one or two approaches. The prevalence approach estimates the cost of a disease in a given year. The incidence approach estimates the lifetime costs of cases diagnosed in a given year. The incidence approach is more useful as calculations give a baseline against which the benefits of new interventions can be assessed, but the approach is more demanding in terms of data and requires estimates of disease progression. The majority of studies are prevalence approaches.

What do cost of illness studies measure?

Ideally, three types of costs are defined.

1   Direct costs form the cornerstone of cost of illness studies and reflect costs incurred by the healthcare system such as drugs and hospitals. However, only since quite recently have direct costs been available with any degree of accuracy within the NHS.
2   Indirect costs measure the economic burden of lost production due to morbidity or premature mortality. There remains a lack of consensus in this area as to the best way to measure productivity losses and whether earnings are a

correct measure of productivity. Due to the problems of calculating indirect costs, it has been suggested that direct and indirect costs should be reported separately in studies. This area is discussed in more detail in Chapter 9.

3   Intangible costs represent the costs of pain, suffering or reduction in quality of life. As it is difficult to allocate a monetary value to this area, intangible costs are usually ignored.

Payments of welfare benefits are not usually included. This is because they represent transfer payments that are used to redistribute income and as a result, there is no societal cost associated with them.

There are a number of methodological difficulties with undertaking accurate cost of illness studies. Due to the high resource demands of the studies themselves, results must be extrapolated from small samples and often illnesses may overlap. For example, it may be difficult to identify and allocate relevant costs where patients have coexisting disease such as diabetes and ischaemic heart disease. Figure 5.1 shows a typical cost of illness study in the mental health sector.

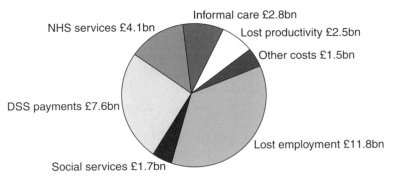

Figure 5.1:   The annual cost of mental illness in England. An example of a cost of illness study that includes social security payments.[3]

An alternative approach to valuing the burden of an illness is the willingness to pay approach. This attempts to measure what society would be prepared to pay to avoid the problem, but there are many methodological problems that limit the usefulness of this technique.

Can cost of illness studies help decision makers?

Cost of illness studies offer an alternative perspective on the importance of diseases compared with other epidemiological indicators, such as morbidity and mortality, and are being used increasingly by pharmaceutical companies to emphasise the importance of a product area. Prevalence studies can provide a

---

Box 5.1:   Features of cost of illness studies

Advantages of cost of illness studies
- They tell us how much society is spending on a disease.
- They identify the different components of cost and the size of the contribution of each sector in society.
- They can help to highlight funding priorities and areas where inefficiencies may exist.
- They can help to identify areas for research priority.

Problems with cost of illness studies
- Costs can be difficult to measure accurately and calculations are likely to be overestimates.
- High cost of illness areas are not necessarily amenable to treatment approaches.
- Simply identifying an area of high expenditure does not provide enough information to suggest inefficiency and should not automatically take precedence for further scrutiny.
- Even if conditions are treatable, expected savings may not arise. For example, certain capital investments will continue to be required and disinvestment may not be possible.

---

baseline against which new interventions can be assessed but due to excessive resource requirements this approach is rarely used. Cost of illness calculations can also help to determine research priorities (Box 5.1).

However, there is a danger that policy makers may be misled by this approach and its importance remains contested among health economists.[4] If these studies are used to allocate resources, it does not necessarily follow that benefit will follow. Allocating priorities on the basis of economic burden also runs the risk of overlooking many important areas of need where there are no economic consequences. For example, foot problems in the elderly would not show up on any cost of illness league table, but chiropody services enhance quality of life of this client group at low cost.

Other economic approaches to burden of illness

Health economists are also involved in measuring indicators of disease burden that are not described in monetary terms. The disability adjusted life year

(DALY) has emerged as a global measure of the burden of disease and is an indicator of the time lived with a disability and the time lost due to premature mortality. It is used to assist in setting health service priorities, to identify disadvantaged groups and to target health interventions. The calculation of DALYs is quite complicated and reflects the number of premature years of life lost combined with the years of disability weighted for age and adjusted to accomodate the fact that disability in the future is valued less than in the present!

- The duration of time lost due to premature mortality is estimated.
- The reduction in physical capacity due to morbidity is measured using disability weights. Disability weights are degrees of incapacity or suffering associated with different non-fatal conditions. Six disability classes measuring the extent of loss of physical functioning associated with a certain condition are defined ranging from 0 (perfect health) to 1 (death). This value is multiplied by the number of years with the disability.
- A value of time lived at different ages is calculated using an exponential function which reflects the dependence of the young and the elderly on adults (i.e. there is a weighting for age that discriminates against the young and the old).
- Finally, DALYs over time are discounted at 3%.

It was estimated that the world's population lost 2,480,237,000 DALYs in 1990 (Figure 5.2). This calculation that seeks to reduce the complexities of global suffering into a single figure may offer us some insights about health economics rather than the state of the world! Perhaps a more useful insight using this approach is that 10% of the world's health research budgets are spent on areas that account for 90% of global disability.

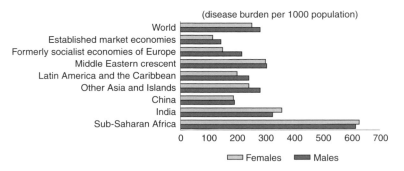

Figure 5.2:   The global burden of disease expressed in DALYs.[5]

Conclusion

Many illnesses create a burden for patients, their families and society. Cost of illness studies aim to quantify this burden by expressing it in monetary terms by itemising, valuing and summing the resources that the condition utilises. They offer an alternative perspective on the importance of diseases compared with other epidemiological indicators such as morbidity and mortality.

Health economists stress the fact that if this approach is used to allocate resources, it does not necessarily follow that benefit will follow or that resources will be used efficiently. Allocating priorities on the basis of economic burden also runs the risk of overlooking many important areas of need where benefit can be gained from simple interventions.

References

1   Rice DP (1994) Cost of illness studies: fact or fiction. *Lancet.* **344:** 1519–20.
2   Byford S, Torgerson D and Raferty J (2000) Cost of illness studies. *BMJ.* **320:** 1335.
3   Patel A and Knapp M (1998) Cost of mental illness in England. *Ment Health Res Rev.* **5:** 4–9.
4   Drummond M (1992) Cost of illness studies: a major headache? *Pharmacoeconomics.* **2(1):** 1–4.
5   Murray C and Lopez (1996) *The Global Burden of Disease.* Volume 1. World Health Organization, Harvard School of Public Health, and the World Bank, Geneva.

CHAPTER 6

The challenge of integrating health and social care: the economist's perspective

Martin Knapp and Ann Netten

The development of primary care trusts offers opportunities for integrating health and social care budgets. However, in many areas, the two cultures are very different and will inevitably pose a number of problems for decision makers. This chapter highlights the challenges of integrating health and social care from an economic perspective and the difficulties of undertaking economic evaluation in this area.

Key points
- Due to the interplay of health and social care on people's welfare there is a policy emphasis on developing closer links between these two sectors.
- Unlike healthcare, there is a highly developed mixed economy in social care with an emphasis on purchaser dominance.
- A rigorous research culture is less well defined in the social care sector and there are endemic problems in the identification of suitable measures of outcome.
- The current moves to integrate health and social care, underestimates the potential difficulties that arise from cultural differences in the two sectors.

Chapter sections
- **Social and health care – the policy context**
- **Social care and economics**
- **The mixed economy in social care**

- Outcome conceptualisation and measurement in social care
- Problems with the research culture
- Conclusion

Social and health care – the policy context

The government has laid out a long-term programme which signals progressively closer links between health and social care provision.[1] Due to the scale and high costs of continuing care of vulnerable people, and particularly older people, the emphasis has been on joint investment plans between primary care groups and trusts and the social service departments of local authorities. While the benefits of partnership are now widely accepted, there are a number of barriers to effective team working and integration which arise from different organisational cultures. Economic insights can facilitate this integration, but the current structure of social care offers a number of challenges to economists.

Social care and economics

The pervasive challenge of scarcity gives economics its universal relevance as much in social care as in healthcare. However, there are particular issues in social care that generate demands for economic insights that are in many respects quite distinct. These include the structure of the mixed economy, the nature of the outcomes of social care and the culture of research. This chapter focuses on these three themes in a UK context. First, however, it is important to be clear what is meant by social care and how it relates to health and healthcare.

What is social care?

In the introduction to *Modernising Social Services*[1] the role of social services is broadly defined as making 'provision for those who need support and are unable to look after themselves'. There are many and varied reasons why these needs for long-term social care arise, but psychological, emotional or physical impairment of some sort is usually a root cause. The objective of healthcare interventions is to prevent, cure or mitigate impairment and disability or, at the very least, maintain ability at as high a level as possible. Social care, on the other hand, is concerned with managing impairment or reducing its effects on peoples' daily lives, such as helping people with personal care tasks or fostering social integration. This does not necessarily mean doing things for people, but ensuring that key aspects of personal welfare are attended to.

What are these 'key aspects of personal welfare'? This depends to some extent on the age and circumstances of the individual. Recent work on developing a measure of social care outcome for older people identified five key domains: food and nutrition, personal care, social participation and involvement, safety, and control over daily life (Box 6.1).[2] For younger age groups meaningful daily activity might also have been included. For children and families yet further domains would be relevant, including family preservation and personal development (in many dimensions).

Box 6.1:   Some key aspects of personal welfare

- Food and nutrition.
- Personal care.
- Social participation and involvement.
- Safety.
- Control over daily life.
- For younger age groups meaningful daily activity.
- For children and families – family preservation and personal development (in many dimensions).

The overlap between health and social care

Due to the complex interplay of factors that affect personal welfare, cause and effect are often not clear. High level needs in these areas of life are associated with situations where there are likely to be physical or health consequences of continuing unmet need. For example, social isolation has been found to be associated with higher levels of morbidity and mortality among older people.[3,4] Behavioural problems in children, if not adequately responded to, can lead to a wide range of social problems in adult life, imposing high costs on health, education, social care and especially criminal justice agencies.[5]

It is in just such areas that health and social care responsibilities have been closely linked or, indeed, overlapped in the past. (For example, both health and local authorities employ occupational therapists.) The current policy emphasis on breaking down the boundaries between health and social care, evident in the NHS Plan,[6] is therefore not new, but reflects longstanding concerns that services addressing such intimately related aspects of people's welfare should work together to achieve the best outcomes. Thus, for example, rehabilitation will be most successful when both health and social care roles are integrated.

The mixed economy in social care

The mixed economy is the collection of arrangements involving the public and independent sectors, for the provision, purchasing and governance of services. This mixed economy is quite different in social care compared with healthcare in the UK, and in a historical context could be seen as more developed. Most residential and domiciliary services for older people, for example, are delivered by private or voluntary organisations, with the state's provider role having declined rapidly over recent decades. There is also quite substantial funding from service users, whereas most NHS healthcare is free at the point of use. Charitable organisations and volunteers have contributed proportionately more resources of money and time in social care than in healthcare.[7] Perhaps the biggest difference, however, is that social care is populated by real markets, where there is a variety of private, voluntary and public providers, and a substantial proportion of care is purchased by individuals in addition to the state. The vast majority of healthcare operates through quasi markets, with NHS organisations acting as purchasers and providers of care.

As noted earlier, social care comprises a wide variety of services, supporting a range of client groups, and the associated mixed economies can be rather different. Here, we focus on services for older people, which account for the lion's share of social care expenditure. We identify the providers and purchasers of care and examine the commissioning and governance frameworks within which they operate.

Providers of social care

There are four main provider sectors:

- the state sector
- the private sector (for profit)
- the voluntary sector (non-profit)
- the informal sector (carers).

The state's provider role is declining in most markets, as convincingly illustrated by residential care (Figure 6.1). The rapid waning of the public sector has been accompanied by a yet more rapid waxing of the private sector, as the

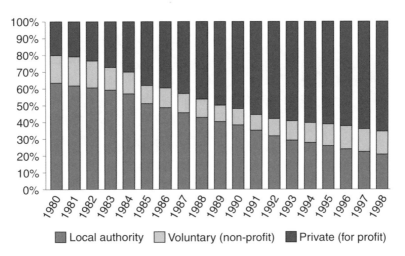

Figure 6.1:   Residential care for older people – residents supported by local authorities.

voluntary sector's market share has been squeezed. The trends in other service areas (domiciliary and day care, particularly) may be less dramatic, but are in the same direction and raise just as many questions and challenges. The private sector comprises thousands of very small businesses – often family affairs running a single facility, with owners expressing a mix of professional, empathetic and profit-oriented motives[8] – and a few large corporate providers. The corporate sector's market share has recently been growing especially fast.

Alongside the formal providers of services sits the largest set of providers – the 'informal sector' of family and other individual care givers. There are now approximately 5.7 million carers in Great Britain, three-quarters of whom provide care to older people.[9] A small proportion of these carers provide highly intensive support and personal services to dependent older people, with nearly one million carers providing co-residential care.[10] In the field of social care there is wide acknowledgement of the key roles played by informal carers, who are both consumers and providers of care. However, economic evaluation of informal care input lags behind that of formal services, and in the field of health-care the practical and economic importance of this sector has only recently started to be recognised.

Purchasers of social care

The largest purchasing source for social care remains tax-based funding, with an increasingly large proportion chanelled to voluntary and private providers through contracts. Charitable funding remains important in some fields,

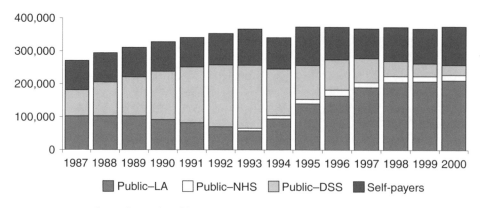

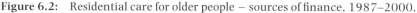

Figure 6.2:   Residential care for older people – sources of finance, 1987–2000.

although proportionately less so than for much of the last century. There are very few incentives to take out social care insurance.

A second important trend in this area has been the shifting funding balance from the social security budget to local authorities. Prior to the full implementation of the 1990 legislation, many older people were able to enter residential or nursing home care and have their fees paid by the department of social security; funding was means-tested, but not needs-related. In other words, anyone wishing to enter such a facility, and finding a facility willing to admit them, could do so. This made the market financially very attractive to private (and voluntary) sector providers, and made government ministers very concerned about uncapped social security expenditure. The 1990 Act transferred state funding responsibility to local authority social services departments, giving much more control over the admission of (publicly funded) people into residential care by ensuring that needs were first assessed. Figure 6.2 shows how the balance of funding changed as a result – with the implementation date of April 1993 marking the beginning of most significant change. The proportion of residents who are entirely self-funded remained fairly constant, but these people add an important dynamic to what is (analytically and politically) a most interesting market.

Governance arrangements

Purchasing and providing may be the most readily identified and regularly discussed dimensions of a mixed economy, but it is their interactions – the transactions or connections between purchasers and providers – which produces the most pertinent elements. The generic economic term for these interactions is governance, and refers to the institutions, rules, regulations and protocols that govern stakeholders in undertaking transactions. Governance examples include the hierarchical structures in public organisations that directly fund their own in-house services, market based mechanisms (such as contracting out), private purchasing of independent services and state support for informal carers. Governance is manifested most clearly through commissioning arrangements.

Commissioning

Commissioning arrangements are more than just the funding links between purchasers and providers. They also include such basic requirements as clarification of organisational objectives and the definition of need, ranging through to the monitoring of contractual relationships and the termination or renegotiation of contracts.

Local authorities are the primary commissioners of social care, and have had to build their commissioning skills from a very low base. Some authorities are beginning to construct long-term relations with their (preferred) providers, although most links remain short term and fairly adversarial, with few 'relational' contracts of the kind advocated by government.[11] The advantage of the latter, provided that the trust inherent in such partnership arrangements is well placed, is that transaction costs can be reduced for both purchasers and providers. It is probably the case that most authorities recognise the attractions of such partnership arrangements, but the majority of them are still only moving slowly towards them.

Contract forms could be seen as quite underdeveloped in social care, with a predominance of spot purchases (on a case by case basis) that leave providers carrying much of the risk inherent in any market. Block contracts that offer a fixed price for a fixed volume of service have only been extensively used so far for day care services. Providers generally prefer block to spot contracts because of the predictability of business that they bring, and in return they may be prepared to accept lower unit prices. On the other hand, purchasers worry that they would risk paying for too many services, and so prefer spot contracts. Cost and volume contracts are still rare, although in guaranteeing a minimum purchase supplemented by cost per case funding they make it easier to build in contingencies and so spread the risk more evenly between purchasers and providers.

Outcome conceptualisation and measurement in social care

Outcomes represent the ultimate benefits to service users. These are difficult to measure, so for commissioning of services and monitoring contracts the focus has often been on outputs or intermediate outcomes, such as quantities of services (e.g. bed days). These are only distantly related to outcomes, so that there are increasing pressures to work towards outcome based contracting. Similarly, in economic evaluation there is a concern with measuring the benefits of services in an accurate and comparable way.

Problems with developing a single measure of outcome

In the field of health economics, the primary drive has been to establish a single global measure that reflects the utility gain of those in receipt of treatment across a wide variety of individual circumstances and interventions. The advantage of this approach is that the benefit gained and cost of that benefit can be compared across different branches of healthcare. However, this approach loses information about other dimensions of outcome, making it problematic for social care, which (unlike healthcare) is characterised by a multiplicity of outcomes, with no simple overarching concept such as 'health-related quality of life' to summarise them. For example, Qureshi and colleagues[12] distinguish between maintenance (meeting basic physical needs), process (a sense of being treated with respect) and change (improving confidence and skills).

Moreover, as social care is not about saving lives, there has not been the historical consensus that 'life years gained' represents a reasonable starting point for assessing outcome. Therefore, there has been no natural progression from 'life years gained' to quality adjusted life years gained, as in health economics. The only 'utilities' that most social care professionals would think about in their daily work are the gas, electricity and water supplies that are cut off when vulnerable clients with chaotic or impoverished lives fail to make their regular payments.

Problems with perspective

There is also the issue of perspective. A family perspective is often fundamental – with children and family services it would be a major mistake only to think about the welfare of the child; indeed 'family preservation' is an aim in its own right. Services for older people are often provided with the express aim of relieving carers in addition to providing support for the direct service user. Not only are outcomes of social care relevant for a range of 'stakeholders', but the interests of these stakeholders may be antagonistic. For example, an older person may prefer to be cared for at home, while for a carer the burden may be such that they would prefer the older person to enter a care home. Perhaps partly because of these issues, the global concept of 'utility' has not been accepted in social care to the same extent as it has in healthcare.

Equity concerns

There are other challenges facing the decision maker seeking to build policy or practice on evidence about outcomes, and also facing the researcher trying to construct such measures. As with healthcare, there is an important societal concern about the welfare of worse off members of society (a 'caring externality'). There is the issue of compulsion – some interventions (such as taking a child into the care of the local authority) are forced upon recipients. If coercion is not the issue, there might still be the contested nature of many decisions. Some – perhaps many – outcomes are intangible; yet users are often unable to express their views, but equally are unable to easily move to another provider.

As a result of some of these difficulties, economic evaluations in the field of social care have tended to identify ranges of outcome measures and used multivariate analyses to link them to costs. The advantage of this approach is a more indepth understanding of the effect of an intervention and its resource implications. The disadvantages are making comparisons across different studies and lack of information about the relative importance of these outcomes to service users or society at large. The recently developed OPUS-SC measure[2] goes some way to overcoming these problems. It incorporates domains central to publicly funded social care of older people across all care settings, and weights them to reflect the preferences of older people, resulting in a utility index that reflects levels of met need, or maintenance outcomes in Qureshi's framework.[12]

Problems with the research culture

It is clear from this discussion of outcome conceptualisation and measurement that there are many and interesting differences between health and social care in regard to economic evaluation. Indeed, the research 'culture' is noticeably different between the two fields. Social work education and the training of social care managers includes much less training in research methods than does medical education. Moreover, although the social care professions endeavour to build their training and practice on solid evidence bases, compared to healthcare there is a much smaller volume and a less robust quality available to them. The issues about outcome measurement have been dealt with above. The are two further problems in the research area outlined below.

Problems with research methodology

An important cultural difference is the rarity of, and quite widespread antagonism towards the randomised controlled design in social care. Few social care researchers have ever been involved in a randomised trial and few openly or actively pursue such a design. Some branches of the social sciences have historically favoured qualitative approaches, which seek to capture the complexities of the social environment.

Problems with 'willingness to pay' and 'willing to accept'

As the majority of users of public social care services are in the lowest income decile, these services are funded by the state only after a means test, and user charges for higher income clients have been so controversial,[13] 'willingness to pay' carries quite different and (to many people) somewhat alarming connotations. It raises the spectre of charging vulnerable people for services that are fundamental to the achievement of a quality of life that is still very modest.

In these contexts, all evaluators – not just economists – face difficulties. In social care the demand for an evidence base is weaker, it is more particularistic (for example in its rejection of some research designs) and it is much less well developed. Many health economists would probably claim to enjoy an ambivalent relationship with their clinical colleagues and with health service managers – sometimes seemingly barely tolerated because cost effectiveness is a 'necessary evil'. For social care economists the challenge of establishing legitimacy is all the greater.

Conclusion

Social care shares many features with healthcare, although in this chapter we have focused on areas of difference. One important difference discussed here is in relation to the structure and development of a mixed economy. Markets are real in social care, only 'quasi' in health – there is a highly developed mixed economy with a long history of non-state involvement in provision, alongside a buoyant private payers' market. There is also a vastly different balance of power today between purchaser and provider. In social care the purchasers dominate providers, whereas in healthcare it has historically been the reverse, although increasingly the aim is for purchasers and providers to work in partnership. Payments for care from different sources, including private individuals, are quantitatively larger and politically more troublesome in social care, as vividly illustrated in the funding debate concerning long-term care.

Another pertinent difference between health and social care is in the nature of outcomes – how they are conceptualised and measured. Social care users are, often by dint of their very needs in many cases, poorly placed to play the role of active, informed consumers; and there are multiple dimensions of need and multiple stakeholders to take into account.

The third area where the experiences of health and social care diverge is in the culture of research. Randomised controlled trials are not widely accepted as appropriate ways to gather evidence in social care, utility has not established a foothold yet in outcome measurement, willingness to pay is regarded with suspicion, and generally there is a much lower level of commitment to building an evidence base.

At the primary care level, there are proposals to merge social and healthcare budgets, and certainly widespread recognition of the need to improve their coordination. The cultural, governance and outcome conceptualisation issues addressed in this chapter represent some of the associated challenges for health economists and commissioners as they seek to capitalise on the opportunities that interagency working offer.

References

1   Department of Health (1999) *Modernising Social Services*. Department of Health, London.
2   Netten A, Ryan M, Skatun D *et al.* (2002) *Development of a measure of social care outcome for older people*. PSSRU Discussion Paper 1690, Report to the Department of Health.
3   Fratiglioni L, Wang H-X, Ericsson K, Maytan M and Winblad B (2000) Influence of social network on occurrence of dementia: a community based longitudinal study. *Lancet*. **355**: 1315–19.
4   Seeman T, Kaplan G, Knudsen L, Cohen R and Gurlnik J (1987) Social network ties and mortality among the elderly in Alameda county study. *Am J Epidemiol*. **126**: 714–23.
5   Scott S, Knapp MRJ, Henderson J and Maughan B (2001) Cost of social exclusion: anti-social children grown up. *BMJ*. **323**: 191–4.
6   Department of Health (2000) *The NHS Plan*. Cm 4818. The Stationery Office, London.
7   Kendall J and Knapp MRJ (1996) *The Voluntary Sector in the UK*. Manchester University Press, Manchester.
8   Kendall J (2001) Of knights, knaves and merchants: the case of residential care for older people in England in the late 1990s. *Soc Policy Admin*. **35(4)**: 360–75.
9   Rowlands O (1998) *Informal Carers*. The Stationery Office, London.
10 Pickard L, Wittenberg R, Comas-Herrera A, Davies B and Darton R (2000) Relying on informal care in the new century? Informal care for elderly people in England to 2031. *Ageing Soc*. **20**: 745–72.

11   Knapp MRJ, Forder J and Hardy B (2001) Commissioning for quality: ten years of social care markets in England. *J Soc Policy.* **27:** 283–306.

12   Qureshi H (1998) *Overview: outcomes of social care for older people and carers.* Social Policy Research Unit, University of York, York.

13   Audit Commission (2000) *Charging with Care.* Audit Commission, London.

CHAPTER 7

A principal–agent perspective on clinical governance

Russell Mannion and Huw Davies

An important feature of current health policy is the emphasis on clinical governance – an interlocking framework of policy initiatives and institutions to improve quality and accountability of clinical care. There is concern that the resources invested into the many facets of clinical governance may not be commensurate with the benefits to the health service that are incurred, but evidence is not as yet forthcoming to address this issue. This chapter does not aim to review the problems of economic evaluation in the area, but offers some economic insights using a principal–agent framework perspective on these new arrangements. This analytical model uncovers some of the key tensions that lie at the heart of clinical governance policies.

Key points
- Clinical governance reflects a move away from professional regulation to more explicit frameworks for monitoring and improving quality.
- The clinical governance agenda is analysed using the principal–agent framework.
- Difficulties arise in the principal–agent relationship when there exists between the two parties both asymmetries of information and incongruent objectives.
- Two broad strategies are available for overcoming the principal–agent problem – checking and trusting.
- For the satisfactory development of clinical governance there will have to be a balance between checking and trusting.

Chapter sections
- **Introduction**
- **The nature of clinical governance**

- The principal–agent economic framework for analysis of clinical governance
- Measurement and monitoring of agent performance
- The role of trust
- Conclusion

Introduction

Turning up the heat on clinical governance

Managing healthcare has often been likened to working in a goldfish bowl; high visibility, sharp political sensitivities and intense media interest means much decision taking happens under a glare of publicity. This impression intensified during the 1990s, which saw the emergence of many calamitous accounts of apparent failures in healthcare. These ranged from concerns over healthcare quality and performance (most traumatically in paediatric cardiac surgery services in Bristol), through issues of consent (e.g. the harvesting of children's body organs at Alder Hey and elsewhere), to numerous 'professional malpractice' cases (of which Harold Shipman was only the most notorious).

At the same time, the UK Government was committing itself to substantial injections of real-term cash growth over the first few years of the new millennium. This policy commitment was accompanied by a considerable anxiety that such investment should reap tangible service improvements in both quantity and quality. Thus, considerable policy energy has been directed at setting frameworks that both encourage quality improvement and ensure efficient use of resources. These frameworks are what constitute 'clinical governance'.

Clinical governance in context

Clinical governance can be interpreted narrowly as the arrangements demanded of provider units (for example, acute trusts, and primary care groups or trusts) in order that they can demonstrate quality and accountability in clinical care. It is these arrangements that will be inspected by the newly formed Commission for Health Improvement (CHI).

More broadly, the emphasis on clinical governance might be thought of as the interlocking policy initiatives and institutional apparatus put in place for controlling and directing the behaviour of clinical staff and the institutions where they work. In addition to CHI these include:

- the National Institute for Clinical Excellence and the National Service Frameworks which provide the standards
- the Performance Assessment Framework and National User Surveys, which monitor progress
- those agencies which are charged with maintaining professional standards, traditionally the Royal Colleges and the General Medical Council and now joined by the National Clinical Assessment Authority.

Analysing clinical governance using the principal–agent framework

There is concern that the resources invested into the many facets of clinical governance may not be commensurate with the benefits to the health service that are incurred. This chapter does not aim to review the problems of economic evaluation in this area, but offers an economic perspective using a principal–agent framework (*see* Chapter 3). It uncovers some of the key tensions that lie at the heart of clinical governance policies. Before embarking on such an analysis, we first examine in a little more detail the nature of clinical governance arrangements demanded of healthcare provider organisations such as NHS trusts.

The nature of clinical governance

Until very recently the quality of NHS clinical services has been the responsibility of a self -regulating medical profession. However, with the publication of the consultation document *A First Class Service: quality in the new NHS* the government introduced the concept of clinical governance and announced that, for the first time in the history of the NHS, lines of responsibility for clinical quality would be integrated with the normal systems of NHS accountability. *A First Class Service* defined clinical governance as 'A framework through which NHS organisations are accountable for continuously improving the quality of their services and safeguarding high standards of care by creating an environment in which excellence in clinical care will flourish.'

Clinical governance has become the key vehicle for continuously improving the quality and accountability of NHS clinical services. It places with healthcare managers, for the first time, a statutory duty for quality of care on an equal status with more traditional areas of managerial responsibility such as finance and productivity. Although many of the core elements of clinical governance are hardly new, the latest arrangements represent an attempt to coordinate and reassemble existing routines to ensure that NHS clinical services are continuously improved.

Box 7.1:   The key components of clinical governance

- *Clear lines of responsibility and accountability for the overall quality of clinical care.* Chief executives are now given ultimate responsibility for assuring the quality of services provided by their organisations. They are also responsible for arranging formal reporting systems and procedures for monitoring quality and clinical performance.
- *A comprehensive programme of quality improvement activities.* This covers a range of mechanisms including: an obligation on clinical staff to participate fully in external audit programmes; engagement with evidence based practice; compliance with national service frameworks; and participation in continuous professional development.
- *Clear policies aimed at managing risks.* These include mechanisms that promote self-assessment to identify and manage risks and the development of effective procedures for the systematic reduction of risk.
- *Procedures for all professional groups to identify and remedy poor performance.* Mechanisms include critical incidence reporting, new complaints procedures, and structures to support professional staff reporting concerns about colleagues' conduct and performance.

Taken together, these new arrangements comprise a comprehensive set of interlocking tactics and supporting initiatives for strengthening clinical accountability and driving up quality (Box 7.1). Whether the clinical governance arrangements will prove successful is ultimately an empirical question. However, in this chapter we set out a simple conceptual framework that can be used to help guide some of the key decisions concerning the development of clinical governance arrangements in the NHS.

The principal–agent economic framework for analysis of clinical governance

This section uses the economic framework of principal-agent theory to explore some of the key issues relating to the design of clinical governance arrangements in the NHS. First though, a brief explanation of principal–agent analysis itself. This has been reviewed in more detail in Chapter 3.

Principals and agents

In all but the least complex of economic systems, it is necessary for an individual or organisation (the principal) to delegate some activities to an agent, who is expected to accomplish these activities at the principals' behest. Thus, in our treatment of clinical governance, the principals are service managers (clinical or non-clinical) within a healthcare organisation who are held accountable for quality and clinical performance. The agents are doctors and other healthcare professionals whose work effort is intended to deliver acceptable levels of quality and performance.

Asymmetry of information and incongruence of objectives

Difficulties arise in the principal–agent relationship when there exists between the two parties both asymmetries of information and incongruent objectives. Where information asymmetry exists (i.e. the principal does not have complete information about an agent's actions and performance), there is a possibility that agents may misrepresent their competence or mislead the principal about their performance. In healthcare for example, this may arise because of the technical nature of the work – clinicians invariably know more about their own actions and consequent outcomes than managers. Problems in the relationship may also arise when principals and agents have divergent aims and objectives. In the NHS for example, hospital managers may view balanced budgets as a priority, whereas clinicians may seek to maximise health benefits for patients.

Solutions to the principal–agent problem: checking and trusting

In a situation where objectives between principal and agents are compatible, even where information asymmetry exists, then there are few problems because the agent will behave in the way the principal wishes them to act. Similarly, if objectives differ between the two parties, but there is an absence of information asymmetry (i.e. there exists reliable and timely clinical performance information), again, there are few problems because in theory the principal is in a position to assess performance and hold agents to account for this. However, in complex organisations, such as a hospital, where outcomes are often difficult to monitor and powerful professional groups seek to pursue their own agendas, there is the potential for both information asymmetries and incompatible objectives to coexist.

Two broad strategies are available for overcoming the principal-agent problem – checking or trusting. Policies can be pursued that reduce the level of information asymmetry by investing in the development of data systems – such as clinical outcome indicators – which can be used to measure and monitor an agent's performance. A second option open to principals is to foster a greater congruence of goals between agents and themselves – such a situation may arise, for example, when principals and agents enjoy a relationship of mutual trust. We now explore the roles of monitoring and trusting in the development of clinical governance systems.

Measurement and monitoring of agent performance

Gathering information on the actions and performance of agents is one way of overcoming the principal–agent problem. Indeed, the collection and publication of clinical outcome data are key to current policy to improve performance in the NHS. It is also clear that providers require high quality information if they are to identify deficiencies in practice and respond accordingly. Therefore, a policy of investing in high quality information may have much to recommend it. However, using performance information such as clinical outcome indicators as mechanisms for strengthening accountability and improving quality has a number of limitations as well as the potential to induce a range of unintended and dysfunctional consequences. Some of these drawbacks are now outlined.

Interpretation difficulties

In order to make assessments of clinical activity it must be possible to attribute poor recorded performance to poor actual performance. In reality, however, it is often difficult to establish such a causal link because of the many intervening factors that serve to weaken the link between actual practice and measured performance. Box 7.2 shows some of the main areas of interpretation difficulty. These issues make assessment of clinical performance somewhat problematic, and mean that great care should be exercised when interpreting variations in measured performance.

Box 7.2:   Areas of difficulty when interpreting performance data

- Clinical indicators based around administrative data sets are commonly found to be incomplete and replete with inaccuracies.
- Variations in case-mix between provider organisations may be the reason for different outcomes rather than differences in clinical performance. Although various risk adjustment models have been developed to take into account differences in case-mix, such models do not represent an exact science and can easily under or over adjust for patient risk factors. Moreover, risk adjustment models will always be incomplete as they can only adjust for known prognostic factors.
- Provider organisations may have little influence on some indicators (e.g. readmission rates) which may depend more on the performance of external agencies such as local social services departments.
- Not all aspects of clinical behaviour and performance can be captured adequately by quantitative indicators. For clinical areas that defy simple quantification, qualitative information transmitted via a range of informal channels and soft intelligence networks may be more timely and provide richer information than 'hard' data collected for official purposes.
- The number of cases observed might severely limit the conclusions that can be drawn because of chance variability. This is a particularly prevalent problem when considering health outcomes.

Dysfunctional consequences of performance measurement

The increased use of clinical performance measures within the new clinical governance arrangements certainly has potential for securing major improvements in the performance of NHS organisations. However, the increased use of performance measures may bring with it the danger that unintended and potentially dysfunctional consequences might arise.[1] If 'what gets measured gets attention', then we can at least expect that organisations and individuals will apply additional effort in those areas where they are measured. This may indeed be appropriate, or it could in turn reflect an inappropriate concentration of effort with consequent neglect of other (unmeasured) areas. Other potential and unwanted effects might include, for example, short termism and suboptimisation to the detriment of overall performance, and a disinclination to innovate.

At the extreme, when measures are used which can bite, gaming, misrepresentation or fraud are all possibilities. The key to successful clinical performance measurement, therefore, is to maximise the beneficial consequences of performance measurement while seeking to minimise adverse effects. A number of strategies might be used to achieve this. These include:

- involving staff at all levels in the development and implementation of performance measurement schemes
- retaining flexibility in the use of performance indicators, and not relying on them exclusively for control purposes
- keeping the performance measurement system under constant review
- maintaining careful audit of the data.

The role of trust

For all the benefits of a measurement approach, full verification of all agent actions and their consequences is simply not possible in any except the most trivial of relationships. Indeed, closing the 'information gap' between agents and principals reflects only one way of dealing with the potential pitfalls of the agency relationship. The second, and more often neglected, approach is to attempt to reduce misalignment between principals and agents in their respective objective functions. This involves a move away from checking and an acceptance of the need for trust.

The necessity of trust

It is not just the quantity of activity that needs checking that poses the problem; it is the variety and complexity of the activities in healthcare that makes checking an incomplete solution. Given the diversity and immeasurability of much of healthcare, health service managers and purchasing authorities cannot hope to check every aspect. For example, formal contracts between principals and agents (e.g. the contracts between health purchasers and NHS trusts) cannot hope to specify in entirety the service desired, and so principals must trust that the aspects unspecified will still be delivered and be delivered well. The inevitability of incomplete monitoring means that principals also need to trust that the unmeasured aspects of performance do not become neglected and degraded. Therefore, although trust may not always be openly acknowledged, almost all principal–agent relationships involve at least some trust as a backdrop to more explicit arrangements. There may also be merit in devising strategies aimed at fostering trust.

What is trust?

Trust is the subjective assessment of the probability of action regardless of monitoring.[2] That is, principals are placing trust in their agent when they come to a judgement that the agent will perform appropriately even when their performance remains unmeasured. Thus trust is a response to the presence of uncertainty and risk which also implies a level of choice – we can choose to trust or we can choose to use other means to encourage action. Trust without an element of choice is merely hope or dependency. Trust acts as a form of social lubricant, facilitating transactions that would otherwise not be possible or economic. If we can trust, then many of the costly overheads of relationships between principals and agents (transaction costs) are obviated. (For further consideration of the implications of transaction costs *see* Chapter 8.)

Building sufficient trust to allow the reduction of transaction costs may not, however, be cost free. It may involve a substantial investment of time and some sunk costs (e.g. building a reputation as a basis for future trust can involve committing resources now for uncertain future benefit). Attempts to build trust may also open up organisations to significant risk of exploitation (i.e. not all attempts to build trust will succeed and those that fail may incur extensive costs).

Balancing checking and trusting

Despite more general societal concerns over falling levels of social trust, at least some of New Labour's policies in the NHS are predicated on the existence of trust between different parts of the health service.[3] For example, a move away from competition and towards partnerships signifies a tacit acceptance that trust matters. In addition, empirical work in the wake of the UK Government's 'Community Care' reforms showed that – in the absence of firm data – reputation and trust were central to the operation of the community care market.[4]

Of course, checking and trusting are not independent – they interact in ways which are not yet clear. There is, however, some evidence that actions which imply a lack of trust (such as performance related pay) may actually diminish performance by displacing intrinsic motivations.[5] However, contexts when this will occur are largely undetermined. Use of performance indicators, especially when published, can certainly imply a lack of trust in professionalism,[6] and may thus impact deleteriously on performance. Further, it is not yet apparent whether trust exists within organisations that are high performers because they are high performers, or whether trust can of itself lead to improved performance. That is, the direction of causality for any associations found between trust and performance is unsettled.

Thus, the crucial relationship between trust and performance is in urgent need of clarification.[7] Despite the upsurge of interest in trust over recent years, and a more explicit recognition of its role within and between well functioning organisations, much remains unclear. Trust may be efficient in many circumstances because of reduced transaction costs compared to checking. In other circumstances it would be foolhardy. The downside of trust is the potential for unchecked inadequate performance or naked opportunism.

Conclusion

Principal–agent theory provides one useful way of analysing new clinical governance arrangements, yet it is not without its limitations. Obviously the model represents a considerable oversimplification – not least because, within healthcare, there are multiple and overlapping relationships that could be modelled in this way.[8] Interactions between these may be nontrivial. Further, the framework contains within it assumptions that top-down managerial authority is the best way of allocating resources and exerting organisational control. This may go against the grain of much of healthcare, where overall direction (and performance) often arises more from an accretion of activity from independent actors. Nonetheless, the framework does succeed in highlighting both the potential and the pitfalls of attempts to redress two key asymmetries: asymmetries of information and misalignment of objectives.

A second key finding to emerge from a principal–agent analysis is that trust is an unavoidable part of the fabric of almost all such relationships. What this means for effective systems of performance management and clinical accountability, however, is not yet clear. Nonetheless, issues of trust cannot be ignored just because they are difficult. A headlong rush for the obvious benefits of checking may be misplaced. What is needed is a thorough analysis of both the costs incurred and the benefits reaped that arise from both systems of checking and strategies of trusting.

Management theorists have sometimes conceptualised agents as either having an inherent dislike of work and, therefore, needing to be controlled and coerced to achieve objectives, or as being intrinsically well motivated and committed and, therefore, in need of support and guidance rather than control. In truth of course, agents may be either of these, neither, or even both – depending on context.[9] To some extent, each conceptualisation is likely to be a self-fulfilling prophecy; strategies of control which assume either set of characteristics will tend to confirm the stereotypes in agents subjected to these regimens. Clearly, economic perspectives on governance issues in healthcare will need to incorporate these softer issues if they are to provide adequate descriptive, predictive and prescriptive models.[10]

References

1 Smith P (1995) On the unintended consequences of publishing performance data in the public sector. *International J Public Admin.* **18**: 277–310.

2 Gambetta D (1988) *Trust: making and breaking co-operative relations.* Blackwell, Oxford.

3 Goddard M and Mannion R (1998) From competition to co-operation: new economic relationships in the National Health Service. *Health Economics.* **7**: 105–19.

4 Mannion R and Smith P (1997) Trust and reputation in community care: theory and evidence. In: P Anand and A McGuire (eds) *Changes in Healthcare: reflections on the NHS internal market.* Macmillan Press Limited, London.

5 Frey B (1997) *Not Just For the Money: an economic theory of personal motivation.* Edward Elgar, Cheltenham.

6 Davies HTO and Lampel J (1998) Trust in performance indicators. *Qual Health Care.* **7**: 159–62.

7 Mannion R and Davies HTO (2001) *Reader's Guide to the Social Sciences.* Fitzroy Dearborn Publishers, London.

8 Propper C (1995) Agency and incentives in the NHS internal market. *Soc Sci Med.* **40**: 1683–90.

9 Davies HTO, Mannion R and Marshall MN (2001) Treading a third way for quality in health care. *Public Money and Management.* **21(2)**: 6–7.

10 Goddard M, Mannion R and Smith P (1999) Assessing the performance of NHS trusts: the use of hard and soft information. *Health Policy.* **48**: 119–34.

CHAPTER 8

Transaction cost economics

Ray Robinson

In the old style NHS, a 'command and control' management hierarchy decided what services were needed and how they should be delivered. The internal market reforms of the 1990s decentralised decision making by introducing a division between purchasers and providers of services. In this system the concept of transaction costs – that is, the costs of buying and selling services – became important. This focus has strong relevance for deciding upon how health services should be organised and for making judgements about the reforms contained in the current NHS Plan.

Key points
- Transaction costs are costs incurred in buying and selling goods and services.
- These costs which had not previously been incurred in the old style NHS became relevant with the introduction of the quasi or internal market in the NHS and continue with the current contractual relationships.
- The present government believes that there is a strong case for moving away from market type relationships and organising the commissioning and provision of care within a more hierarchical, integrated system.
- If higher transaction costs result in better services, they may be worth incurring.
- Transaction costs are difficult to measure and political claims over the advantages of different healthcare systems must be treated with caution.

Chapter sections
- **Introduction**
- **Economics of transaction costs**
- **Transaction costs – what is the evidence?**
- **Conclusion**

Introduction

Transaction costs are the costs incurred in buying and selling goods and services. The concept came to prominence in the NHS following the introduction of the internal market in the early 1990s when contracting between purchasers and providers led to a range of costs that had not been incurred previously in the old style NHS. Within the primary care sector, GP fundholders, GP fundholding consortia and total purchasing pilot sites all drew heavily on the contracting system in order to secure service improvements from providers.[1] Indeed, it was the level of transaction costs thought to be associated with GP fundholding (and other aspects of the internal market) that provided the New Labour government with one of the main reasons for replacing it with its own set of reforms.

Although these reforms retain the formal separation between purchaser and provider organisations, transaction costs are expected to be reduced through a greater degree of integration between purchasers and providers and reliance on long-term service agreements rather than short-term contracts. *The NHS Plan* mentions savings of £1 billion from lower management and transaction costs through the latest reforms.

To investigate the substance of these claims, this chapter examines transaction costs in theory and in practice. It starts by considering the ways in which

---

Box 8.1: Some definitions

- A *contract* is a formal agreement between purchasers and providers that specifies the services that will be provided and the terms on which they will be provided.
- A *service agreement* performs the same basic function as a contract but is intended to be less formal and to run over a longer period of time, thereby reducing transaction costs.
- A *market* is any arrangement by which buyers and sellers come together. It may be a physical location or virtual (e.g. stock markets).
- An *internal or quasi market* is the term coined for market type arrangements that were introduced into the public sector during the 1990s.
- A *managed market* is the term used to refer to markets that are subject to regulation in order to ensure that important social objectives (e.g. fairness) are not neglected.
- A *transaction* occurs when a service is bought and sold.
- *Transaction costs* refer to the costs incurred in buying and selling goods and services.

Table 8.1:   Minimum contracting requirements of the Department of Health as an example of contract elements[2]

- Nature and level of service provided
- Price
- General or specific population characteristics
- Criteria for admission, discharge and referrals
- Waiting times
- Quality measures
- Information that the parties will make available to each other
- Methods of monitoring the contract
- Methods of billing, authorisation and settlement

economists have analysed transaction costs. This is followed by a discussion of the ways in which transaction costs have been measured in practice in primary care. Finally, ways of organising NHS activity that can be expected to minimise transaction costs in the future are discussed. Some definitions are provided in Box 8.1, and an example of contract elements is shown in Table 8.1.

Economics of transaction costs

Transaction costs are the focus of a branch of economics known as the 'new institutional economics' (NIE). This approach maintains that organisational structures will reflect the need to minimise transactions and other management costs. If the costs of buying and selling goods becomes too great, there will be an incentive for firms to seek to reduce them by internalising what were external market transactions within a hierarchical managed structure. Thus management decisions within an integrated organisation replace market transactions.[3,4] There have been many examples of this process in industry generally, such as oil companies taking over petrol stations and brewers taking over public houses!

The theory goes on to specify those characteristics of a market that will tend to favour hierarchical control.

- *Bounded rationality*: The volume of information that market decision makers need to take into account in order to make fully rational decisions is often simply too great for them to deal with. Put another way, there is information overload. In these circumstances, a market will not necessarily produce an efficient outcome.
- *Opportunism*: When information requirements are large – and particularly when one party to a transaction has more information than another – there

is a danger that buyers and/or sellers may operate opportunistically in order to further their own ends. That is, deceit and other forms of dubious ethical behaviour may take place. To ensure that this does not happen, it will often be necessary to rely on elaborate monitoring systems designed to prevent opportunistic behaviour. These add to the costs of operating a market system.

- *Asset specificity*: When one party is tied into a transaction because the majority of their physical and human capital is geared to business with a particular purchaser or provider, there is clearly a danger that they will be susceptible to opportunistic behaviour. The concept of 'hold-up' – whereby the party with the stronger bargaining power imposes unreasonable terms on the more vulnerable party – is a well known consequence of asset specificity. Fear of hold-up can also make providers reluctant to invest in capital equipment and thereby lead to suboptimal levels of investment.

What is the relevance of these factors for the NHS? Put simply, many economists have argued that contracting within the internal market was characterised by bounded rationality, opportunism and asset specificity. For example, purchasers were required to assemble large amounts of information on alternative providers' prices and the quality of care supplied. Unfortunately, information systems were often nonexistent, or failed to provide accurate and timely information. Assessing the multidimensional aspects of the quality of care involving structures, processes and outcomes posed particular problems.

All of these factors inhibited fully rational purchasing decisions. While a general commitment to NHS values might be relied on to prevent the more extreme aspects of opportunism, hard pressed NHS managers certainly faced incentives to 'game' the system through data manipulation and other strategies in order to survive in a competitive environment. Finally, many providers were geared to meeting local needs and did not really have the scope for switching their assets to alternative modes of production. Equally, purchasers' needs for local access frequently meant that there was no real alternative to the local provider.

Taken together, it can be argued that the existence of these characteristics provides a strong case for moving away from market type relationships and organising the commissioning and provision of care within a more hierarchical, integrated system. Within such a system, managerial edicts replace market transactions and can be expected to economise on transaction costs. Certainly the move away from short-term contracting and towards longer-term service agreements is consistent with this view. Before any judgement is made about the wisdom of this move, however, it is worth considering more closely the ways in which transaction costs arose in the internal market. To anticipate our conclusions, it may be that transaction costs have not been reduced as much as was expected and that some offsetting benefits – such as greater choice for purchasers and patients – have been jeopardised.

Transaction costs – what is the evidence?

Despite the frequent reference to the heavy costs of contracting during the 1990s, remarkably little systematic evidence is available on the subject. One notable exception was a study of transaction costs carried out as part of the national evaluation of the total purchasing pilot sites.[5]

Fifty-three first-wave total purchasing pilot (TPP) projects were established in England and Scotland in April 1995. These sites had the potential to purchase virtually all of the hospital and community health services used by their resident populations and, as such, engaged in extensive contracting activities.[6] These sites were also the subject of an independent, national evaluation. As part of the national evaluation, the level of transaction costs that they incurred were examined at a sample TPPs.[5] To do this, the researchers identified four categories of transaction costs.

- *The costs of search and information*: These covered the costs incurred acquiring information about providers' prices, quality of care and other aspects of their services.
- *The costs of negotiation and contracting*: These covered the time and other costs involved in negotiations with providers and writing the contracts for the supply of services.
- *The costs of monitoring and enforcement*: Provider performance needed to be monitored over time to ensure that it complied with the contractual agreements on activity, prices and quality. Moreover, in those cases where providers failed to meet contractual agreements, actions needed to be taken to either ensure compliance or agree variances from the original terms of the contract.
- *The costs of coordination and organisation*: Because the individual GP practices that were grouped together in a single total purchasing pilot site were required to agree on the allocation of a shared budget, considerable time and effort needed to be devoted to coordinating activities of individual practices.

In considering these categories of costs, it is worth noting that the fourth category – the costs of coordination and organisation – is not a conventional transaction cost as defined by the new institutional economics (NIE). The counterparts of these costs in NIE are the internal managerial costs incurred within an organisation. These are usually held to be less than would be incurred through external transactions. In the case of TPPs, however, the organisation could be more properly defined as a network. As such, a range of extra costs of coordination is incurred in addition to the conventional ones considered in NIE. This point is worth emphasising as the same costs may well persist in the New Labour healthcare system.

What did Posnett's study[5] show? First, it raised the question of why there was such a wide range of transaction costs. When expressed as a cost per registered patient, the mean transaction cost was £2.83 with a minimum of £1.42 and a maximum of £4.18. These transaction costs were in addition to the internal management costs of each TPP which also amounted to about £2.82 per capita. Why were the costs of transactions at the highest cost TPP double those at the lowest cost project? Further analysis by the researchers sought to identify the reasons for these cost variations. The size of the TPP might be thought to be one determining factor. In fact, size can be expected to affect costs in two opposing ways. On the one hand, economies of scale can be expected to lead to reductions in costs per capita, as the size of the organisation expands and fixed management costs are spread over a larger population. Set against this tendency, however, as an organisation increases in size, the costs of coordination tend to become greater. The opposing directions of impact of these factors was probably the reason why the researchers found no systematic relationship between the size of a TPP and its level of transaction costs. In fact, the only relationship to emerge from this part of the study was a positive correlation between self-reported success rates and the size of management costs.

Second, inspection of the separate components of total costs indicated that the costs of searching and acquiring information (43%) and significantly the costs of coordination (42.9%) were the two largest components. Third, although the study was confined to only 3 years, there was no indication that the level of transaction costs fell over time as TPPs became more used to the system of purchasing. Finally, none of the costs stated were related to the benefits that were incurred. Higher levels of transaction costs may have been delivering more effective and better quality services.

Conclusion

Alongside the perceived inequity of GP fundholding (and its variants such as total purchasing), the heavy transaction costs that it was felt to impose on the NHS was one of the main reasons for the New Labour government's decision to abolish the scheme. The above discussion suggests that there are strong theoretical reasons to expect heavy transaction costs, but that rigorous empirical evidence on the subject is scarce. Nonetheless, the government's preferred strategy has been to create larger scale primary care groups/primary care trusts (PCGs/PCTs) and to require them to establish stable collaborative arrangements with their providers. Long-term service agreements are expected to replace shorter-term market contracts.

To what extent will this system reduce transaction costs and result in a more efficient system of organisation? A full answer to this question can only be provided through careful measurement of current and future levels of transaction costs. Nonetheless two provisional judgements can be made, based on the experience of the last 10 years.

First, reductions in transaction costs – broadly defined – may be much smaller than the government expects. The reason for predicting this outcome is that the considerable task of coordinating individual practices' actions will be even greater within the larger, extended networks of PCGs/PCTs (comprising conscripts and not volunteers as in earlier forms of primary care based commissioners) than was the case in TPPs. Furthermore, as the empirical work outlined above showed, these coordination costs constituted a major part of total transaction costs. The costs of contracting *per se* were actually rather small.

Second, economic evaluation should be based on an assessment of the full range of costs and benefits of alternative courses of action. The analysis so far has concentrated on only the cost side. If the benefits of decentralised, primary care based commissioning – defined in terms of service improvements obtained through the leverage of contracting – are sufficiently great to offset additional transaction costs, the higher cost system may nonetheless be more efficient.

Both of these messages point to the need for the careful collection of data on the costs and benefits of the different ways that commissioners and providers work together. This is necessary to ensure that cost effective options for the provision of services are chosen and not those based on ideology, fads or fashions.

References

1   Glennerster H, Matsaganis M and Owens P (1994) *Implementing GP Fundholding: wild card or winning hand?* Open University Press, Buckingham.
2   Department of Health (1989) *Contracts for Health Services: operational principles.* HMSO, London.
3   Williamson O (1975) *Markets and Hierarchies.* Free Press, New York.
4   Williamson O (1985) *The Economic Institutions of Capitalism.* Free Press, New York.
5   Posnett J, Goodwin N, Griffiths J *et al.* (1998) *The Transactions Costs of Total Purchasing.* National evaluation of total purchasing pilot projects. Working paper. King's Fund, London.
6   Robinson R, Robison J and Raftery J (1998) *Contracting by Total Purchasing Pilot Projects.* National evaluation of total purchasing pilot projects. Working paper. King's Fund, London.

Section 3

Aspects of economic evaluation

Economic evaluation forms the bulk of health economists' work and provides the core of this book. It is the area that will be of most relevance to healthcare managers and practitioners and offers an explicit framework within which costs and benefits of alternative healthcare interventions can be compared.

Before the introduction of fundholding, there was little information on NHS costs at any level. The importance of the purchaser/provider split was to illuminate this fact but did little to improve it. However, although there still remains some way to go, NHS cost information is getting more accurate. In Chapter 9, Ann Netten and I explore some basic costing principles and concepts that should be used in a costing exercise.

Health economists are at pains to stress that costs should not stand alone, but must be related to the benefits that their investment produces. In Chapter 10, I wade out alone into deeper water to explore how outcomes can be measured and used from the perspective of the health economist. Although here I take the party line, as a practitioner I am aware of the difficulties of capturing relevant outcomes in a complex dynamic system such as healthcare.

To undertake economic evaluation, studies must be undertaken that compare intervention costs to their benefits and Chapter 11 highlights how this can be done and some of the difficulties that are encountered. However, the information that economic studies deliver is rarely in a form that is helpful to end users. It is often incomplete and may need interpretation by experts. Chapter 12 reviews how economic evaluation can be presented and used by those who make resource decisions in healthcare.

CHAPTER 9

Costing interventions in healthcare

Ann Netten and David Kernick

An accurate assessment of costs is an important part of any economic evaluation.

How costs are derived and combined will depend on the assumptions that have been made in their derivation. It is important to be clear what assumptions have been made and why in order to maintain consistency across comparative studies and prevent inappropriate conclusions being drawn. This chapter outlines some costing concepts, principles and problems.

Key points

- Cost information is necessary for planning, management, performance measurement and economic evaluation.
- Until recently, we had very little idea of the cost of things in the NHS. The situation is improving but there is still much room for improvement.
- There are a number of costing rules which help to maintain consistency across studies.
- Always think carefully about the perspective or viewpoint of a costing exercise – this will determine which costs to count.
- There is a lack of consensus in some areas of how costs should be calculated, statistically manipulated and reported.

Chapter sections
- **Introduction**
- **Approaches to cost estimation**
- **Basic costing concepts**
- **Some basic costing 'rules'**
- **Conclusion**

Introduction

Accountants view costs as financial expenditures necessary for the provision of activities and are not concerned with the value that is placed on the expenditure. Economists emphasise the importance of value and see costs occurring when a productive activity takes place that necessitates the use of scarce resources that could be used for some other purpose. They seek to value costs in terms of this benefit foregone. This concept can be important in terms of what is costed when evaluating services. However, in practice, due to the difficulties of identifying and valuing the opportunity cost, costs are usually derived from the sum of the financial expenditures necessary for the production of the item under consideration.

Costs are a fundamental building block of any economic evaluation. Until quite recently, there was a paucity of accurate cost information across the NHS. The growth of interest in cost measurement has been driven by the need for cost information for planning, management and performance measurement, in addition to formal economic evaluation.

How costs are derived and defined will depend on the assumptions that have been made in their derivation. The *New NHS Costing Manual**** sets out the principles and practice to be applied in the NHS, and data supplied by NHS trusts are used to compile a national reference cost index that allows providers to compare costs on a consistent basis.[†] This national reference cost database provides a first step in describing and understanding variations in costs between NHS suppliers, but there remain serious drawbacks in the quality and coverage of the data used, and much of the variation in costs may be statistically insignificant.[1] There is currently no evidence to suggest that reference costs encourage more efficient production of healthcare.[2]

Many gaps still remain where there is a pressing need for accurate cost information and uniformity. For example, at a time of increasing partnership between health and social care agencies, guidance available to cost health and social care resources are very different, based as they are on different histories and organisational requirements.

This chapter outlines some costing concepts and issues that need to be considered when undertaking an economic analysis in the field of health and social care.

Approaches to cost estimation

There are two principle approaches to cost estimation. In the top-down approach, total resource use is divided by activity. For example, from knowing

---

* www.doh.gov.uk/pub/docs/doh/manual5.pdf (not for the faint hearted)
† www.doh.gov.uk/nhsexec/refcosts

Box 9.1:   The bottom-up costing process

Stage 1 – Identify the activity (e.g. the GP consultation).

Stage 2 – Describe the elements of the activity to be considered (e.g. GP time, administrative backup, capital overheads, ongoing education).

Stage 3 – Identify the unit costs of each element.

Stage 4 – Estimate the quantity of each element needed to undertake the activity to give the total service cost.

---

how much expenditure is allocated to GP services and knowing how many consultations GPs provide each year, the cost of each consultation can be calculated. However, this approach may overlook many important resource inputs and there are often problems in linking resources to activity. This is particularly the case where resources are used jointly to produce a number of activities (for example, in hospitals). A more accurate approach is a bottom-up estimate, which identifies and attaches a value to all the relevant resources associated with a particular activity (Box 9.1). Current guidance in the *New NHS Costing Manual* aims to improve cost estimates by reconciling the results of these two approaches.

Basic costing concepts

Opportunity cost

When resources are limited, someone's gain is somebody else's loss. When measuring resources in economic terms, the objective is to identify the opportunity

---

Box 9.2:   Valuing the opportunity cost of a GP's time

Consider the cost of a GP increasing consultation time by an extra hour. The GP may work the same number of hours but reduce services provided in other areas so the opportunity cost is the value of the services displaced. Alternatively, the working week may be extended so the opportunity cost is that of the GP's leisure time. In practice, the most appropriate estimate of the cost will depend on the context of the evaluation and the perspective of the exercise.

---

cost – the value of the best alternative foregone in order to provide that service (Box 9.2). Identifying the opportunity cost can be difficult. Although the principle is important and should always be borne in mind, in most cases estimates are based on the expenditure on relevant inputs. This is legitimate in that the expenditure could have been spent on purchasing 'the best' alternative. Problems arise where there is no clearly identifiable expenditure (for example, *see* costs below of informal care).

Classifying costs

Traditionally costs have been classified as direct or indirect. Direct costs represent the resources consumed by a service and associated events (Table 9.1). For example, direct costs associated with primary care include GP time, practice nurse time, drugs and capital costs arising from equipment and buildings.

Indirect costs may be tangible – productivity losses or inputs from carers, or intangible – loss of leisure, costs of pain, suffering, uncertainty or death. As indirect costs do not have a market value, costs allocated to them are known as 'shadow prices'. Deriving these values demonstrates the difficulty in certain areas of costing. For example, costs associated with loss of economic activity are likely to form the major component of indirect costs, but there remains a lack of consensus over how they should be derived.[3] From a societal viewpoint, work loss may have a direct effect on gross national product although the contribution towards economic performance will vary between patients. This approach assumes that the economy is working at maximum efficiency, but in many cases the loss of a productive unit will have no effect on output. Losses may be made up when returning from short-term absence and for longer periods, the patient can be replaced by an unemployed worker.

Greater difficulties arise when evaluating indirect costs for which there is no market price.[4] For example, 'non-wage' time may consist of leisure time or non-market productive activity, such as housework, and can be an important component in many clinical studies. An approach which is based on trade-off judgements that are made between possible alternatives with cost as a factor

Table 9.1: Types of costs that are identified by health economists

Direct costs	Costs associated directly with a healthcare intervention (e.g. GP salaries, drug costs)
Indirect costs	Costs associated with reduced productivity due to illness, disability or death
Intangible costs	The cost of pain and suffering occurring as a result of illness or treatment

values non-wage time at approximately 25% of work rate.[5] An alternative approach is to use the domestic wage rate as a 'shadow price' for the lost opportunity of domestic activities.[6]

In many cases, non-wage and work time may overlap, and difficulties may arise in separating these elements when illness and medical interventions have implications for both. For example, a patient attending a hospital outpatient session in the afternoon may make up his lost employment by staying extra time on return to work, in which case the cost of attendance is his/her leisure time. Clearly, costing exercises are rarely as straightforward as one might expect!

Theoretically, the cost of intangibles such as pain and suffering, loss of leisure and death should be valued and included in an economic analysis, as these constitute a loss to society. Not surprisingly these costs are difficult to value. One approach is to identify how much society is willing to pay to avoid them. An alternative approach is to capture intangibles through measures of outcome. For example, the value of a quality adjusted life year (QALY) should encompass elements of intangible losses. Where willingness-to-pay approaches are used to identify intangible loss, it is important to be aware of potential double counting (i.e. valuing intangibles in both the inputs and outcomes of an economic evaluation).

An alternative classification particularly for economic evaluation is health service costs, non-health service costs and non-resource costs (Box 9.3). While transfer payments do not constitute an opportunity cost to society, they do represent public expenditure and as such are of interest in some economic evaluations. This is particularly the case when there are long-term care implications.

Box 9.3:   An alternative description of costs

Health service costs
- Direct costs of the whole intervention including the broader health service costs.
- General illness costs – costs of undergoing therapy for other illnesses while being treated for the intervention in question which may or may not be unrelated.
- Future health service costs – these may arise as a result of individuals living longer because of the intervention and can be due to related or unrelated diseases.

Non-health service costs
- Costs incurred by other public sector budgets (e.g. social services). Including this element will identify cost shifting that may occur.
- Patients' travel costs and other expenses.

- Informal care costs – the costs incurred by carers including unpaid time.
- The opportunity cost of patients' time associated with receiving treatment.
- Productivity costs associated with morbidity and mortality.
- Future non-health service costs.

Non-resource costs
- These are often known as transfer payments – flows from one societal budget to another (e.g. Social Security payments). As there is no net gain to society, they involve no resource consumption and are excluded from an economic evaluation.

Marginal costs

Most decisions in health are not concerned with whether a service should be provided or not but whether to expand or contract an existing service. For this reason, health economists advocate the use of marginal costs rather than average costs. For example, the average cost of N consultations will be the total cost of GP services divided by N, and the marginal cost will be the cost of the $(N + 1)$th consultation. As most costs will have fixed and variable elements, in the short run marginal costs will differ from average costs (Table 9.2).

However, we are usually interested in long run costs as these reflect the full costs to society of an intervention, including fixed costs. For example, if the evaluation is concerned with a way of working that implies a greater need for GP time, then if this is to be introduced more GPs will be needed. To have more GPs we need to train and equip them and provide premises, all resources that are 'fixed' in the short term, but have long-term resource implications.

Table 9.2:   An illustration of the difference between total, average and marginal costs for a day case surgical procedure. The cost of £2000 represents the fixed overheads of the unit

Number of patients	Total cost (£)	Average cost (£)	Marginal cost (£)
0	2000	–	–
1	2500	2500	500
2	3000	1500	500
3	3250	1083	250
4	3300	825	50

Capital costs

Capital costs are fixed in the short term and are associated with premises or equipment that are not used up in the process of providing a service.

Costs and time

Ideally, an economic study should be long enough to cover the period over which all types of resources including capital facilities can vary.

Discounting future costs

In many cases, an intervention will incur costs in the future and competing interventions may have different patterns of expenditure. In general, we prefer to incur costs later rather than sooner and in economic terms this is known as time preference. To quantify this difference and enable costs to be integrated and compared within a single time frame, evaluations that extend over a period of more than a year should discount future costs in order to express total costs in present value terms (Table 9.3). Costs should be evaluated at the end of each year and discounted at the prevailing rate using the formula:

Present value $= \sum C_n/(1 + r)^n$

Where

$n =$ year under consideration
$C_n =$ costs in year n
$r =$ discount rate

The Treasury sets the discount rate for the public sector which is currently 6% p.a.[7]

Table 9.3:   An example of actual and discounted costs of two competing interventions, which incur costs over 3 years

	Year 1	Year 2	Year 3	Actual total cost	Discounted total cost
Intervention A	50	100	200	350	321
Intervention B	200	100	50	350	338

Costs changing with time

Unit costs may not always be available within the same time frame. For example, cost data may only be available for a particular year prior to a study. Where necessary, unit costs must be adjusted by an NHS-specific inflator. These are published annually in *The Unit Costs of Health and Social Care Report* (*see* resources at the end of the chapter).

Which costs should be counted – defining the perspective of an exercise

The perspective of a study will dictate which costs to count. The perspective of the individual patient, the GP practice, the purchasing authority, the NHS or society in general, can all be considered, and different answers may be obtained for each approach (Table 9.4). Health economists generally advocate a comprehensive societal perspective measuring all costs regardless of who incurs them. More limited perspectives may mask the fact that costs are simply being shifted elsewhere rather than being saved.

Presenting comprehensive data in a disaggregated form allows an analysis to be undertaken from different viewpoints, allowing the needs of key decision holders to be met.

Table 9.4:   Think carefully about the perspective about a costing exercise – different perspectives give different answers

What does a GP Cost?[8]	
Perspective	*Cost*
GP practice	£21/hour
Health Authority (includes central overheads)	£53/hour
NHS (includes training costs)	£69/hour

Allowing for uncertainty – the role of sensitivity analysis

Given the problems associated with cost estimation, it is important to identify sources and assumptions when reporting cost studies, and wherever possible test the sensitivity of any conclusions drawn to any assumptions made across the range of cost estimates that are found. Sensitivity analysis allows the outcome of an analysis to be tested over a range of situations likely to be found in practice to determine the robustness of analysis to potential changes in key variables.[9]

Statistical manipulation of cost data

Although the principles of statistical inference are well advanced in the analysis of clinical data, some issues relating to the statistical analysis of economic data remain unresolved,[10] and improvements in the statistical analysis and reporting of data are urgently required.[11] One of the major problems is the conflict in sample size required for adequate power between clinical outcomes and economic evaluations. In most cases, larger trials are needed to detect statistically important differences in economic indices than clinical measures, but usually clinical requirements prevail.

A misleading conclusion can be drawn in the absence of supporting statistical cost data. For example, a relatively small number of high cost events can disproportionally effect overall costs and the ability to detect significant cost differences between interventions. How cost data are best analysed remains a matter of debate.[12]

Some basic costing 'rules'

Studies undertaken at different times or places may not be comparable unless standard costing procedures are used. For example, a recent review of twenty studies that derived the cost of a GP consultation[13] found a range of between £3 and £11 depending on the method of costing used. Knapp[14] has identified a number of 'rules' to be used when estimating and using cost information that can help ensure uniformity. For example:

- Costs should be accurately and comprehensively measured to prevent inappropriate conclusions being drawn from a costing exercise. Costs can vary in the way they are valued and combined. There will inevitably be resource implications in obtaining accurate data, but if the conclusions of a study are sensitive to variations in a particular unit cost it should be accurate and all relevant costs included. For example, a meningitis immunisation programme must include not only nurse costs and equipment but also implications for practice administrative and managerial staff in addition to cost implications of attending patients.

- Like should be always compared with like. Care must be taken to avoid drawing inferences from misjudged comparisons. Inappropriate comparison with respect to case-mix is unlikely to be an issue when cost data are generated alongside comparative trials. Problems are more likely to arise from omission of important elements of costs relevant in one context but not another. For example, studies of early hospital discharge should include living costs at home over the study period as hospital costs will include living expenses of an in-patient.
- Costs should never stand alone but always be related to outcomes. It should always be borne in mind that in isolation, cost data mean very little. The cost of a service or intervention should always be considered in relation to the output or benefit it produces.

Conclusion

Deriving costs is not the straightforward exercise it may seem, and concern still remains over the accuracy of cost data within the NHS. How costs are defined and combined should be clearly identified in any economic evaluation, as different approaches may effect the conclusions of a study.

There is no such thing as a gold standard cost estimate. How cost is estimated will depend on the purpose of the exercise. For every study, sources and assumptions should be clarified as far as possible with the aim of enabling end users to adapt the information and substitute better information where or when it is available. Whenever possible ranges of estimates should also be provided. Nevertheless, there are some fundamental principles that will help practitioners, managers and commissioners think a little clearer about the decisions they make.

Resources

- Netten A, Dennett J and Knight J (1998) *The Unit Costs of Health and Social Care Report.* PSSRU, University of Kent, Canterbury – compiles a comprehensive list of unit costs and pay and prices inflation indices which is updated annually. www.ukc.ac.uk/PSSRU/
- Netten A and Beecham J (eds) (1995) *Costing Community Care: theory and practice.* Ashgate Publishing, Aldershot – an in-depth but accessible look at costing principles from the community perspective.
- A comprehensive review of costing in economic evaluation and its theoretical foundations can be found in the Health Technology Programme publications.[15] www.hta. nhsweb.nhs.uk

References

1 Dawson D and Street A (2000) Reference costs and pursuit of efficiency. In: P Smith (ed) *Reforming Markets in Healthcare.* 187–210. Open University Press, Buckingham.

2 Appleby J and Thomas A (2000) Measuring performance in the NHS: what really matters? *BMJ.* **320:** 1464–7.

3 Liljas B (1998) How to calculate indirect costs in economic evaluations. *Pharmacoeconomics.* **13(1):** 1–7.

4 Posnett J and Jan S (1996) Indirect costs in economic evaluation: the opportunity cost of unpaid inputs. *Health Economics.* **5:** 13–23.

5 Fowkes T (1986) The UK Department of Transport values of time project. *International J Transport Economics.* **13:** 197–207.

6 Knapp M (1995) Costing informal care. In: A Netten and J Beecham (eds) *Costing Community Care: theory and practice.* Ashgate Publishing, Aldershot.

7 HM Treasury (1989) *Discounts rates in the public sector.* Circular 32/89.

8 Netten A, Dennett J and Knight J (1998) *The Unit Costs of Health and Social Care Report.* PSSRU, University of Kent, Canterbury.

9 Briggs A, Bland R, Cheetham J *et al.* (1994) Uncertainty in the economic evaluation of healthcare technologies: the role of sensitivity analysis. *Health Economics.* **3:** 95–104.

10 O'Brian B, Drummond MF, Labell ER *et al.* (1994) In search of power and significance: issues in the design and analysis of stochastic economic appraisals. *Medical Care.* **32:** 150–63.

11 Barber J and Thompson S (1998) Analysis and interpretation of cost data in randomised controlled trials: review of published studies. *BMJ.* **317:** 1195–200.

12 Thompson S and Barber J (2000) How should cost data in pragmatic randomised trials be analysed? *BMJ.* **320:** 1197–200.

13 Graham B and McGregor K (1997) What does a GP consultation cost? *Br J Gen Pract.* **47:** 170–2.

14 Knapp M (1995) Principles of applied cost research. In: A Netten and J Beecham (eds) *Costing Community Care: theory and practice.* Ashgate Publishing, Aldershot.

15 Johnson K, Buxton M, Jones D and Fitzpatrick R (1999) Assessing the cost of healthcare technologies in trials. *Health Technol Assessment.* **3(6).**

CHAPTER 10

Measuring the outcomes of a healthcare intervention

David Kernick

Although information about health service activity has always been available in some form, until recently comparatively little was known about the benefits or outcomes of many of the services provided. The evaluation of outcomes can be seen as part of a wider concern to manage resources more efficiently and improve the quality of services delivered. This development has been reflected in a move away from an overreliance on subjective judgements, where it has traditionally been assumed that doctors know what is best, to a more explicit and technical approach to the delivery of healthcare. This chapter considers how we measure outcomes and where health economists fit in.

Key points
- The measurement of outcomes is part of a wider agenda to monitor and improve health service quality and manage resources more efficiently.
- Health economists use outcomes to compare alternative service or treatment options by relating them to the costs incurred in providing them.
- There has been a shift in emphasis from clinical outcome measures to broader measures based on health related quality of life measurements.
- There still remains considerable debate over conceptual and methodological issues on how quality of life should be measured.

Chapter sections
- Introduction
- Measuring health related quality of life
- Using health outcomes in economic evaluation
- Conclusion

Introduction

Historically, measurement of process or activity such as number of GP consultations or hospital bed occupancy was seen as sufficient to manage the health system, but the outcomes or results of this activity were largely overlooked. Although we now have a whole host of indicators, many of these remain proxies for outcomes (e.g. emergency admissions and readmissions), and may reflect other influences such as deprivation rather than poor quality or inappropriate healthcare provision. Measuring outcomes at a broad level is difficult due to these complexities of cause and effect. Nevertheless, we can aim for a greater degree of accuracy evaluating outcomes for individual interventions.

Over the past 25 years, the health outcome movement has gathered pace driven by three factors:

- a realisation that the evidence base for healthcare activity was limited and the growth of the evidence-based medicine movement
- concern over the wide variation of activity that was found across the National Health Service
- the need to obtain value for money against a background of increasing demands on limited resources.

Information on outcomes is essential if politicians, consumers, commissioners and providers are to make decisions aimed at providing cost effective, high quality care. However, the requirements of economic evaluation are often different from other uses of outcome measurement (*see* Box 10.1).

The outcome movement has been driven by a philosophical approach known as consequentialism – the proposition that the worth of an action can be assessed by the measurement of its consequences (i.e. its outcome). Historically, mortality has been the main outcome measure, but over the past 30 years clinical outcome measures (e.g. blood pressure, renal function, depression score)

Box 10.1:   The principal applications of outcome measurement

- To assist health professionals in monitoring patients' progress.
- To identify benefits of new medical interventions.
- For audit, quality assurance and healthcare contracting.
- To enable epidemiological studies to highlight inequity in health and relate it to population characteristics and health service delivery.
- To facilitate the allocation of limited resources in an efficient manner.

have become increasingly important. This change has reflected the development of medical science and, in particular, the pharmaceutical sector. Although this approach may suffice for many areas, there are a number of problems.

- There may not be a direct relationship between the clinical indicator and final outcome of interest. For example, a drug introduced to reduce abnormal heart rhythms after heart attacks did so successfully, but was found to increase mortality when evaluated over a long period of time.
- The approach is limited to comparisons of interventions with similar outcomes. It is unable to inform decisions between disease groups or healthcare programmes with different outcomes.
- Clinical measures give a very narrow measure of the impact on patients and may give a distorted picture. The objective implied by the measure is not being questioned nor its worth valued. Different stakeholders may have different ideas on what is important and the weights placed on various measures of outcome. For example, one study sought the views of doctors, patients and their partners on the effects of a new antihypertensive drug.[1] The doctors were very satisfied from a clinical perspective; patients expressed some concerns but were happy their doctor was pleased; spouses expressed strong reservations about the impact on the patient's quality of life due to side effects.

The recognition that the personal burden of illness cannot be fully described by clinical measures alone led to the development of health related (or more accurately healthcare related) quality of life measurements. However, despite a huge literature extending across the fields of philosophy, psychology, sociology, medical and health economics, a unified approach has yet to be devised for the measurement of quality of life,[2] and there remains considerable debate over

---

Box 10.2:   Some basic requirements of an outcome measure

- Appropriateness – is the outcome measure appropriate to the question it seeks to address?
- Acceptability/feasibility – can the outcome be readily measured with an instrument (e.g. a questionnaire) that is acceptable to patients and easy to administer?
- Reliability – does the outcome instrument produce results that are reproducible and consistent?
- Validity – does the instrument measure what it claims to measure?
- Responsiveness – does the instrument detect changes over time that matter to patients?

conceptual and methodological issues.[3] In fact, when examined closely, the distinctions between 'health' and 'quality of life' become blurred and the definition issue becomes relegated to a discussion among philosophers which invariably has no satisfactory resolution! Nevertheless, there are some basic requirements for any outcome measure which are shown in Box 10.2.

Measuring health related quality of life

There is no consensus on the definition of quality of life as affected by health. One approach is to assume it to be those aspects of an individual's subjective experience that relate both directly and indirectly to health, disease, disability and impairment.[4] Calman[5] uses a definition of 'the gap between experience and expectation'. This approach helps to explain why patients with severe disability do not necessarily report a poor quality of life. The implication of this definition is that current measures do not take into account expectation and cannot distinguish between changes in the experience of disease and changes in the expectation of health. As both these factors are likely to change during an illness, measures of health related quality of life may be changing continuously! Despite these concerns outcome measures are available and are being used with increasing frequency. Current health related quality of life measures are divided into two main groupings depending on what they try to measure and how they present their findings.

What are we trying to measure? – Disease specific or generic quality of life measures

Measures can be disease specific and include questions that are important to patients with a specific problem, but inappropriate for other patients or the general population (e.g. asthma related quality of life). Alternatively, generic instruments focus on the impact on a patient's life in a more general sense. They have the advantage that they can be used in a variety of settings and allow comparison between different patient groups. They may not be as sensitive to changes in disease status and treatment. (The relative merits of each approach is a subject of hot debate among health economists who argue as if there was a *right* answer for a *perfect world*.)

How are findings presented? – Profile or single score

Health status instruments can be classified according to the type of data they produce. Many instruments yield a profile with scales for several different dimensions that are presented separately as shown in Box 10.3. These aim to cover all the relevant domains of health related quality of life, such as pain and psychological status, and in principle they can be applied across a wide range of diseases to enable comparisons to be made between different patient groups and with healthy populations. The most widely used instrument is the Short Form 36 (SF36).[6]

Box 10.3:   Typical components of a generic, profile quality of life instrument. Each component is scored and presented separately rather than attempting to compress into an overall single index

- Physical function (e.g. mobility, activities of daily living)
- Symptoms (e.g. pain, nausea)
- Psychological well being (e.g. anxiety, depression, sense of control)
- Social well being (e.g. social integration)
- Cognitive functioning (e.g. memory, alertness)
- Role activity (e.g. employment, financial status)

Alternatively, instruments can provide a single score index of health status for all dimensions covered, for example the EuroQol[7] – now known as the EQ-5D. However, even with the broader approach of generic instruments, other sources of benefit and disbenefit that affect health status can still be overlooked.[8] Patients may obtain unmeasured benefit from the process of care arising from such factors as information, reassurance or choice.

Using health outcomes in economic evaluation

Health economists use outcomes to compare treatment options and their costs. Within the formal economic framework, single index measures are required to

Table 10.1:   Types of economic analysis – the analysis takes its name from the outcome that it considers

Form of evaluation	Measurement and valuation of outcomes	Comments
Cost minimisation analysis	Outcomes are assumed to be equivalent – focus of measurement is on costs	Simplest approach but outcomes are rarely equivalent
Cost effectiveness analysis	Natural units (e.g. life years gained, reduction in blood pressure)	Most common approach – limited in terms of questions that can be addressed
Cost benefit analysis	All outcomes valued in monetary units (e.g. valuation of a patient's willingness to pay for a cure)	Rarely used due to difficulties with valuing outcomes in monetary terms
Cost utility analysis	Health state values based on individual preferences (e.g. quality adjusted life years gained)	Increasing in popularity but remains controversial

enable direct comparisons to be made. Health economists argue that it is necessary to attach values to possible outcome states in order to determine what these states mean to people. For example, what are they prepared to give up to receive the benefit? However, although theoretically important, identifying these values is not always possible or practical. Table 10.1 shows how outcomes can be measured in an economic evaluation.

Cost minimisation analysis

In a cost minimisation analysis, the consequences of two or more interventions being compared are equivalent. The analysis therefore focuses on costs alone. In practice, there are few examples of interventions, which produce exactly equivalent outcomes. An example of this type of analysis would be the comparison of two antibiotics, which have the same treatment benefits and side effects.

Cost benefit analysis[9]

In this approach, attempts are made to value all the costs and consequences of an intervention in monetary terms. Although this approach has the advantage of estimating the net benefit/cost to society of a programme or intervention, the data requirements are large and methodological issues around the valuation of non-monetary benefits, such as lives saved, makes this approach problematic.

Cost benefit analyses were the first type of economic evaluation to be developed and adopted the human capital approach to measuring benefits. This sees healthcare as an investment in health making more labour available to the economy, but the ethical and conceptual limits of this framework restricted the development of this approach. An alternative approach is known as 'willingness to pay'. This derives monetary values to outcomes by asking members of the public, patients or other groups about their willingness to pay for the outcome in question. Again, there are many problems that include the issue of whose values should be used, how to give respondents sufficient information to enable informed choice and how to obtain values that are not related to respondents' income. Due to methodological difficulties, this form of analysis is not widely used although a comeback seems to be occurring.

Cost effectiveness analysis[10]

Due to the problems with cost benefit analysis, a simpler approach where common health outcomes are measured in natural units (e.g. reduction in cholesterol, life years saved) has increased in importance. The first studies were published in the late 1960s and now account for the majority of economic evaluations. If an intermediate outcome measure such as blood pressure reduction is used, it is important to ensure that these surrogate measures have some clinical meaning in terms of long-term outcome for patients.

Cost effectiveness analysis is used to facilitate technical efficiency (i.e. achieving a given clinical objective at the least cost or maximising a clinical objective from a fixed sum of money). Its disadvantages are that the worth of an outcome (what it means to people) is not valued, it cannot compare interventions that have different outcomes and it cannot encompass quality of life.

Cost utility analysis[11]

Often it is necessary to compare competing healthcare alternatives that have different outcomes. For example, should resources be directed to hip replacement or coronary artery bypass surgery? Here the main requirement is for an instrument which is applicable to a wide range of conditions (generic), which produces a single index score and encompasses broader issues such as quality of life. A cost utility analysis is similar to a cost effectiveness study except that effects are expressed as measures that reflect the value of ill health years lost.

The concept of utility

Utility is an important concept that we consider here in some detail. Utility was first defined in 1789 by the philosopher Jeremy Bentham as 'that property of an object whereby it tends to produce benefit, advantage, pleasure, good or happiness or to prevent the happening of mischief, pain, evil or unhappiness to the party whose interest in considered'. In economic theory, utility signifies the benefit a person expects to gain from the consumption of goods or services – an indicator of the consumer's strength of preference. Utility is an attribute that motivates us to choose one action over another. It will be a complex function of a number of elements that might include physical, psychological and moral components that we integrate in our minds to form preferences.

A major methodological breakthrough was achieved in the early 1970s with the application of utility theory to economic evaluation which led to cost utility analysis. In health economics, utility reflects the individual's preference for a particular state of well being derived from the consumption of healthcare. For example, if we had three drugs that could cure asthma, diabetes and migraine we might place our utility preferences as diabetes treatment first, asthma second, migraine third. However, this list tells us nothing of the strength of our preferences. For the technical calculations that economic evaluation requires, we need to put a number on this (i.e. we need to quantify our strength of preference for each treatment outcome). Conventionally, a scale of between 0 and 1 is used, and the strengths of each preference for the utility that a healthcare intervention provides will be somewhere along this scale.

Health economists stress the importance of obtaining the value of this preference by methods that reflect scarcity and sacrifice. They argue that just asking someone to place their preference on this scale does not really reflect the true value they put on it. For example, we might ask someone who has 10 years left to live how many years of their life would they trade-off to be relieved of their disease. This will give us preference values for the outcomes of the treatments of the three conditions above, and we now have a way of comparing the outcomes of three disparate interventions. Although that seems simple in theory, behind this approach lies a huge methodological debate.

The most frequently used measure is the quality adjusted life year (QALY). The utility value is multiplied by the number of years in that state to produce the number of QALYs – the equivalent 'years in full health' (Box 10.4).

There are three main approaches to deriving utility that we will now consider. Only the second and third methods are underpinned by formal economic theory. However, the first approach has attractions in terms of practicality.

Box 10.4:   An example of a QALY calculation

A treatment costs £400 and yields 0.8 utility units over each of 5 years against doing nothing.

The cost is £100 per QALY (£400/0.8 × 5).

Preference based approaches

Preference based approaches generate utilities from an array of hypothetical health states derived from population samples. For example the EQ4D presents health states which cover five dimensions (mobility, self-care, usual activities, pain/discomfort and anxiety/depression). Within each of these dimensions there are three possible levels (no problems, some problems and major problems). Respondents are asked to value a single health state in terms of these dimensions and levels. For example, the hypothetical state may have no problems with mobility and self-care, some problems with self-care, no problems with pain and discomfort and major problems with anxiety and depression.

Alternatively, a simple scale measurement can be used which asks patients to place their current health status on a line that goes from 0 (death) to 1 (perfect health). However, these two approaches do not truly assess the value or the utility that the patient would gain from the health state. One way of assessing this value is by ascertaining what people would sacrifice to attain this health state. Drawing on the fundamental economic principles of scarcity and sacrifice, two further techniques are defined.

Time trade-off

The time trade-off method asks subjects to decide how many years of remaining life they would exchange for complete health. For example, if a patient with rheumatoid arthritis had 10 years to live and would be prepared to trade 2 years of their existing life for 8 years of perfect health using a curative drug, the utility gained from the drug would be 0.2 over each year of life.

Standard gamble

The standard gamble asks individuals to choose between living the rest of their lives in their current state or gambling on a cure which if won will mean perfect health and if lost, signify death. The odds are varied until there is indifference between the two events and this probability expresses the individual's preference for their health state. For example, a patient with rheumatoid arthritis is asked to imagine a room with two doors. Going through one will enable life to remain the same. Going through the other will allow a X chance of cure

$(1 > X > 0)$ or a $(1–X)$ chance of death. X is varied until the patient is unsure of which door to go through, and from this the utility can be calculated.

Cost utility evaluation

Many commentators argue that the cost utility approach should be treated with caution and QALYs have been criticised in a number of areas some of which are shown in Box 10.5.

Conceptual and empirical difficulties in cost utility analysis have prevented a rapid proliferation of this approach. For example, a review published in 1992 counted 51 published cost utility studies, most of which were methodologically deficient.[12] A recent update of this review showed an increasing number of studies but continuing problems in their methodological quality. Table 10.2 shows some estimates of cost/QALY for common healthcare interventions. However, QALYs are gaining increasing importance particularly with central

---

Box 10.5: Some concerns with cost utility analysis

- QALYs discriminate against the elderly disabled who have less opportunity of benefiting from an intervention than those more fortunate.
- Should QALYs be corrected for age? Some argue that it is correct to weigh the QALYs for different age groups to reflect their economic contribution or the fact that the elderly have had their fair innings.
- The clinical evidence on which the cost utility analysis is based may be limited.
- Small changes in health status that are important to the patient may not be registered.
- There are methodological problems. Different methods of derivation give different results. For example, many people are 'risk adverse' and will tend to choose the safer option if presented with a gamble.
- There is an assumption that possible outcomes and the probabilities of each outcome are known in advance, whereas in reality this is rarely the case.
- Who should do the rating? Should this be the patient or carers who knows the condition, healthcare professionals or citizens who actually pay for the treatment and are potential patients themselves?
- The cost utility approach overlooks the impact on the quality of life of family and carers.
- Can the complexity of life be reduced into a single unit? Decision makers may be seduced into thinking that by using the cost utility approach, simple solutions are available for inherently complex problems.

Table 10.2:   Some estimates of cost per QALY of competing interventions[13]

Intervention	Cost per QALY (£1990)
GP advice to stop smoking	270
Antihypertensive therapy	940
Hip replacement	1180
Coronary artery bypass graft for severe angina	2090
Kidney transplant	4710
Breast cancer screening	5780
Hospital haemodialysis	21,970

decision-making bodies such as the National Institute for Clinical Excellence (NICE). The fundamental concern, however, is that they measure people's preferences for health states rather than their capacity to benefit from healthcare. This approach inevitably leads to the conclusion that a disabled life has less value than a life without disability and in the US, the QALY has had little impact, as it is seen to violate the rights of disabled people.

To counter some of the concerns with the QALY, a number of other approaches have been developed which are shown in Box 10.6. In general, they differ from the QALY in methodological approach and all have been criticised on theoretical grounds. In practice, they have not found widespread use. (For a comprehensive discussion on the philosophical and methodological problems with the QALY that demonstrates the almost overwhelming complexities of assigning quality of life on a scale between 0 and 1 see www.jiscmail.ac.uk/files/esrc-hrqol/edgar.doc.) Before turning to the subject of cost consequences analysis, some practical examples of the types of economic evaluation already discussed are presented in Box 10.7.

Box 10.6:   Alternatives to the QALY

- Healthy year equivalents – reflects the number of years that could be spent in perfect health compared to the number of years in imperfect health. For example, 10 years of perfect health may be considered as equivalent to 15 years with arthritis.
- Saved young life equivalents – these calculate how many people receiving an intervention would be equivalent to one saved young life equivalent.
- Disability adjusted life years – these combine the expected length of life lost with the adjusted number of years lived with the disability.

Box 10.7:   Practical examples of economic analyses

A cost minimisation analysis – hospital at home versus hospital care.[14] There was found to be no difference in outcomes between patients randomised to care at home or hospital. NHS, Social Services, patient and family costs were measured. Home care could deliver care at similar or lower cost than an equivalent admission to an acute hospital.

A cost effectiveness study – management of urinary tract infection in general practice.[15] The cost and benefits (symptom free days) of seven possible treatment options for urinary tract infection in general practices were considered. The most cost effective strategy was treating clinical presentations with antibiotics, which provided two symptom free days at a cost of £7 per day above a baseline of doing nothing. Incremental cost effectiveness ratios were calculated above this baseline (e.g. adding laboratory culture costs an additional £215 per symptom free day averted).

Cost utility analysis – a study of interferon beta in multiple sclerosis.[16] A study of interferon beta in secondary progressive multiple sclerosis estimated a cost of £1 million per QALY gained and it was suggested that money would be better spent on other ways of improving quality of life.

Cost consequence analysis

A consequence analysis[17] is not recognised as a formal method of economic evaluation. It is a pragmatic framework that has attractions to healthcare decision makers. The rational underpinning of the above methods of economic evaluation has been the belief that the outcomes associated with treatment options can be aggregated into a single measure to facilitate decision making. This simplistic approach has had limited impact to date due to the multiple dimensions of healthcare outputs that include not only effectiveness but tolerability and harm. There may also be more complex considerations for decision makers such as patient opinion, policy contexts, historical precedents and availability of local resources.

An alternative approach is to present costs and outcomes in a disaggregated form, often drawing on different sources. This avoids the need to represent cost/benefit results as a simple ratio, which may be an unrealistic simplification of the healthcare environment. Healthcare decision makers can then apply their own context to the results and use items that are relevant to their particular

Table 10.3:   Results of a cost consequence study of the benefits of a Dermatology Nurse working in general practice,[19] demonstrating a wide range of outcome measures that can be considered

Costs	Benefits
Training costs	Generic quality of life – improved but not statistically significantly against control
Costs of running a dermatology clinic	
Savings in GP consultation time	Dermatology related quality of life instrument – improved but not statistically significantly against control
Prescribing cost implications	
	Change in clinical score – increased statistically significantly against control
	Qualitative data obtained from patients showed considerable value from the clinic
	Qualitative data from GPs and practice staff support initiative – for example, helped to break down skill-mix barriers, led to the introduction of other skill-mix innovations
	Expert opinion judges to be of value (e.g. NHS Beacon Practice award as a result of initiative)
	Facilitated working across primary–secondary interface

situation and time frame. Although cost consequence studies do not fall within the classical health economic framework, in many cases they may be a more attractive option for decision makers, and it has been argued that this approach appears to be the most robust and socially defendable method at this time.[18]

Table 10.3 shows a cost consequence study measuring the impact of a dermatology nurse in general practice, which takes a range of outcome data in addition to evidence from a randomised controlled trial.

Conclusion

Health economic evaluations use outcomes to facilitate the explicit and efficient use of limited healthcare resources by relating the outcomes of interventions to their costs. Within the formal economic framework, single index measures are required to enable direct comparisons to be made. Attempts to measure these health benefits are based on the belief that outcomes alone are not enough and wherever possible, it is necessary to attach values to possible outcome states.

However, no practical, unified approach has been devised to integrate the disparate outcomes of health interventions. What gets measured will depend on the context of the exercise and the agency that sets the evaluation agenda. It has been argued that in some cases measuring the processes of care may be more enlightening than outcomes.[20]

The outcome movement is not without its detractors who claim that it is not possible to condense the complexities of life into a single measure. These concerns and others are explored in some detail in Section 6. For example, there may also be problems obtaining the true preferences of patients who may distort their values if they know that health status measures are being used to influence the allocation of resources. Nevertheless, there is an increasing emphasis on the use of outcomes, and an appreciation of their advantages and methodological problems is essential to all those working in the healthcare sector.

Resources

A comprehensive review of the use of health status measurement in economic evaluation can be found in the Health Technology Programme publications.[21] (www.ncchta.org)

References

1   Jackuk SJ, Brieley H and Jackuk S (1982) The effects of hypertensive drugs on the quality of life. *J R Coll Gen Pract.* **32:** 103–5.
2   Gill TM and Feinstein AR (1994) A critical appraisal of quality of life measurements. *JAMA.* **272(8):** 619–26.
3   Mulldoon M, Barger S, Flory J *et al.* (1998) What are quality of life measurements measuring? *BMJ.* **316:** 542–5.
4   Carr A, Gibson G and Robinson P (2001) Is quality of life determined by expectation or experience? *BMJ.* **322:** 1240–3.
5   Calman K (1984) Quality of life in cancer patients – an hypothesis. *J Med Ethics.* **10:** 124–7.
6   Ware J and Sherborne C (1992) The MOS 36 item short form health survey: a conceptual framework and item selection. *Medical Care.* **30:** 473–83.
7   EuroQol Group (1990) Euroqol: a new facility for the measurement of health related quality of life. *Health Policy.* **16:** 199–208.
8   Ryan M and Shackley P (1995) Assessing the benefits of healthcare: how far should we go? *Qual Health Care.* **4:** 207–13.
9   Robinson R (1993) Economic evaluation and health care: cost benefit analysis. *BMJ.* **307:** 924–26.

10 Robinson R (1993) Cost effective analysis. *BMJ.* **307:** 793–5.
11 Robinson R (1993) Cost utility analysis. *BMJ.* **307:** 859–62.
12 Gerard K (1992) Cost utility in practice: a policy maker's guide to the state of the art. *Health Policy.* **21(3):** 249–80.
13 Drummond M and Maynard A (1993) *Purchasing and Providing Cost Effective Healthcare.* Churchill Livingstone, London.
14 Jones J, Wilson A, Parker H *et al.* (1993) Economic evaluation of hospital at home versus hospital care: cost minimisation analysis of data from a randomised controlled trial. *BMJ.* **319:** 1547–50.
15 Fenwick E, Briggs A and Hawke C (2000) Management of urinary tract infection in general practice: a cost effectiveness analysis. *Br J Gen Pract.* **50:** 635–39.
16 Forbes R, Lees A, Waugh N *et al.* (1999) Population based cost utility study of interferon beta in secondary progressive multiple sclerosis. *BMJ.* **319:** 1529–33.
17 Mauskopf J, Paul J, Grant D *et al.* (1998) The role of cost consequence analysis in healthcare decision making. *Pharmacoeconomics.* **13(3):** 277–88.
18 Eccles M and Mason J (2001) How to develop cost conscious guidelines. *Health Technol Assess.* **5(16):** 4.
19 Kernick D, Reinhold D, Sawkins J *et al.* (2000) A cost-consequence study of the impact of a dermatology-trained practice nurse on the quality of life of primary care patients with eczema and psoriasis. *Br J Gen Pract.* **50:** 555–8.
20 Davies H and Crombie I (1994) Assessing the quality of care. *BMJ.* **311:** 766.
21 Brazier J, Deverill M, Green C *et al.* (1999) A review of the use of health status measures in economic evaluation. *Health Technol Assess.* **3(9).**

CHAPTER 11

Undertaking economic evaluations

David Kernick

To undertake an economic analysis, the benefits of competing healthcare interventions must be related to the resources utilised in their production. This chapter reviews how such studies can be undertaken and some of the difficulties that are encountered.

Key points
- Historically, economic analysis has been driven by the pharmaceutical sector. This has led to an emphasis on economic evaluation alongside a controlled trial.
- The type of economic evaluation takes its name from the benefit that is measured. The approach used will depend on the question that is being asked.
- Complete data will not always be available for an economic exercise and often models will be used, with data where it is available and expert opinion where it is not.
- There remain a number of methodological areas where consensus has yet to be achieved, but guidelines have evolved to ensure compatibility across studies.

Chapter sections
- **Introduction**
- **Undertaking economic evaluations**
- **Which form of economic evaluation should be used?**
- **Some problems to be addressed when relating costs to outcomes**
- **Using models in economic evaluation**
- **Guidelines for economic studies**
- **Conclusion**

Introduction

An economic evaluation provides a framework to compare the benefits and costs of alternative interventions to facilitate choice when resources are scarce. Although there remain a number of methodological problems, economic evaluation offers a useful framework that can facilitate the difficult choices that confront decision makers and ensure that resources are used in an efficient manner.

Previous chapters have considered how costs and outcomes can be measured, but to undertake economic evaluations, studies must relate the benefits of competing healthcare interventions to the resources used in their production. This chapter reviews how economic data can be collected and handled. The following chapter considers how such data can be presented to decision makers.

Undertaking economic evaluations

Methods of evidence generation are viewed as a 'hierarchy' with the randomised controlled trial (RCT) taking precedent over other study designs (Box 11.1). Historically, economic evaluation has focused on the pharmaceutical sector where interventions lend themselves to investigation using the RCT.

However, the primacy of the RCT has been questioned in a number of areas.[1] A controlled trial will not always capture the complex patterns of interactions that are a feature of the healthcare environment. An alternative view would be to match the analytical approach to the complexity of the environment. For example, Hammond[2] has described a 'cognitive continuum' of decision making whereby structured systems can be examined by analytical approaches such as the RCT, but as tasks become less organised, intuition and expert opinion are important.

Box 11.1: The hierarchy of evidence

Meta-analysis of high quality trials
Multicentred RCT
Single centre RCT
Historic control
Case–control
Database analysis
Case series
Expert opinion

Box 11.2:   Some problems of undertaking economic analysis alongside controlled trials

- Randomised controlled trials rarely reflect the environment in which the interventions are to be delivered – patients are usually atypical and experimental time periods are less than those found in practice.
- Statistical power requirements for clinical and economic elements are often different. Clinical considerations usually prevail leaving trials underpowered from an economic perspective.
- Many interventions are already accepted into practice, and it would be unethical to repeat randomised controlled trials for economic purposes.
- There are resource implications when undertaking economic studies, which may not be commensurate with the importance of the question to be answered.

Although health economists are recognising the value of other methodologies,[3] the gold standard is to undertake economic analysis alongside the randomised controlled trial wherever possible (Box 11.2).

Which form of economic evaluation should be used?

Table 11.1 shows the main approaches to economic evaluation which have been reviewed in the previous chapter. The type of economic evaluation used

Table 11.1:   Main forms of economic evaluation

Study type	Measurement and evaluation of consequences
Cost minimisation analysis	Outcomes assumed to be equal – focus is on costs alone
Cost effectiveness analysis	Natural units (e.g. life years gained, reduction in blood pressure)
Cost utility analysis	Health state values (e.g. quality adjusted life years gained)
Cost benefit analysis	Monetary units
Cost consequence analysis (not a formal method of economic analysis)	Multiple outcomes presented in a disaggregated form

will depend on the question that is being asked. Few interventions have identical outcomes and cost minimisation analysis is rarely used. The most common type of evaluation is a cost effectiveness analysis, that aims to provide a maximum output for a fixed cost or a fixed output for the lowest cost. Cost effectiveness studies consider competing interventions in similar clinical areas.

When different interventions are being considered (for example resource allocations between mental health or cardiovascular disease) and there is no common clinical outcome measure, or when decision makers wish to encompass quality of life, a cost utility analysis will be the method of choice. Due to methodological problems of converting all outputs into monetary values, cost benefit exercises have not been widely used.

Some problems to be addressed when relating costs to outcomes

When undertaking economic analyses there are a number of theoretical and practical considerations.

Which comparator?

An economic evaluation compares interventions, and ideally all options should be considered including doing nothing. However, this may not be ethical or practical. In principle, the comparator should be the most cost effective alternative available to enable the opportunity cost to be determined. In practice, it is usually the most widely used treatment, but it should be borne in mind that if current practice is unevaluated, a new intervention may appear to be cost effective when in fact it is not.

Which perspective?

The study perspective determines which costs and, in some cases, which benefits to include in an evaluation.[4] Different results may be obtained from the perspective of the patient, the GP, the PCG/PCT, the NHS or society. A societal perspective incorporates all the costs and benefits regardless of who incurs or obtains them. In practice, it is rare that a societal perspective is undertaken, but more restrictive perspectives may mask the fact that costs have simply been shifted to another sector rather than being saved.

Time horizons

The nature of the problem studied will dictate the time over which an intervention should be analysed, which in many cases will be the duration of a patient's life span. In some cases, the impact of an intervention will only become apparent after a considerable length of time. However, decision makers and researchers need quick results if they are to be acted on and submitted for academic accreditation. In this situation, long-term analysis is only practical on the basis of predictive modelling using short-term primary data.

Discounting costs and benefits

Cost may be incurred and benefits enjoyed at different times when comparing interventions. As we prefer to incur our benefits sooner and costs later (due to the opportunity cost of capital and psychological time preference), these variables must be multiplied by a factor so that they can be evaluated and compared within the same time frame. This is known as discounting[5] and is usually applied to economic trials that last for more than a year. However, there still remains a lack of consensus over the appropriate discount rate particularly for benefits.

Table 11.2 shows the effects of discounting costs and benefits of two treatment options. Although the overall costs and benefits are identical they occur at different times over the 3-year period. Therefore, to bring the analysis to the same time frame of year 1, both costs and benefits that are incurred in the future are reduced by the annual discount rate.

Table 11.2:   Two competing interventions demonstrating the effect of discounting. Without discounting both treatments cost £10,000/QALY. Discounting costs and benefits – treatment A costs £9660/QALY, treatment B costs £10,627/QALY

		Year 1	Year 2	Year 3
Treatment A	Cost	£1000	£1000	£1000
	(QALYs gained)	0.1	0.1	0.1
Treatment B	Cost	£2000	£500	£500
	(QALYs gained)	0.05	0.05	0.2

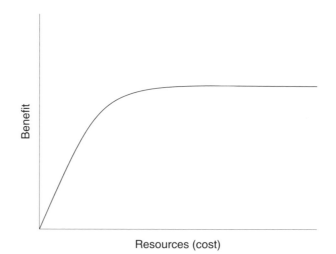

Figure 11.1:   The law of diminishing marginal returns and the importance of marginal analysis. Benefits do not continue to increase in a linear manner as more resources are invested into any healthcare intervention. It is, therefore, important to relate increments in resources invested to the incremental increase in benefits.

Undertaking a marginal analysis

Because the relationship between costs and benefits is rarely a straight line (Figure 11.1), the important measurement is not an average cost per benefit (the total cost divided by the total benefit), but the incremental ratio (how increments in benefit change with increments in costs.) This is known as a marginal analysis.[6] For example, a recent study of cholesterol lowering therapy found that the average cost effectiveness ratio for patients was £32,000 per life year gained, but this average concealed differences in patient subgroups depending on their risk level of between £6000 and £361,000 per life year saved.[7]

The importance of undertaking a marginal analysis should always be recognised, but often benefits cannot be tested over a range of resource investments. If this is the case, an attempt should be made to define the most relevant incremental analysis to perform based on the context of the exercise.

Local validity of economic studies

Most trials evaluate treatments in research environments that may not be representative of routine clinical practice. This can lead to unrealistic estimates of costs and benefits, and decision makers need to be aware of these drawbacks.

Box 11.3:   Relevant questions for local decision makers

- Does it compare the options I am interested in?
- Is the perspective relevant for my circumstances?
- Does it include all the costs and effects that are relevant to me?
- Are the data sources locally relevant?
- Do the costs apply to my situation?
- Have costs and effects been adjusted to reflect differences in timing that may occur?
- Is the comparison between options relevant to me?
- Can I see how uncertainty impacts on the results?
- How relevant to me is the conclusion likely to be?

Ideally, study design should be transparent enough to allow decision makers to insert their own local parameters, but the data and expertise for this exercise are not always available. Box 11.3 shows some questions that may be relevant for local decision makers.

Problems with statistical analysis

Although the principles of statistical inference are well advanced in the analysis of clinical data, some issues relating to the statistical analysis of economic data remain unresolved.[8] One of the major problems is the conflict in sample size required for adequate power between clinical outcomes and economic evaluations. In most cases, larger trials are needed to detect statistically important differences in economic indices than clinical measures but invariably, clinical requirements prevail. A further problem is that a relatively small number of high costs can disproportionally effect overall costs and the ability to detect significant cost differences between interventions.[9]

Currently, the main approach to resolving issues of uncertainty is the use of sensitivity analysis. Sensitivity analysis is a crude but useful means of exploring how sensitive the results of an economic evaluation are across the range of data that may vary. It allows the robustness of results to be tested in light of variations in the values of key variables. For example, if cost estimates are specific to a particular locality, investigators can generalise across the costs found in a number of different sites across the NHS. However, problems can still arise. For example, if 19 out of 20 sensitivity analyses of a study indicate no change in conclusion, this does not mean that the results are statistically significant and there remain difficulties with interpretation of such findings.

Economic evaluation and equity concerns

What is efficient is not necessarily what is fair, and a recent review of the literature on economic evaluation[10] demonstrated a complete neglect of the equity
dimension. The studies surveyed did not provide enough information for
decision makers to make their own judgements about the impact on various
population groups affected by the policy under study.

Some health economists have tried to address these issues by developing an
equity weighted QALY, but there appear to be insurmountable theoretical and
practical problems. Perhaps the best approach is to present information on the
cost implications and benefits in different population groups. Decision makers
can then apply their own values and trade-offs to the choices that have to be
made, taking into account national policy and local considerations.

Using models in economic evaluation

An economic model captures the essence of reality, simplifying relevant issues
to the minimum level while retaining their principal components. Models have
a number of uses in economic evaluation.[11]

- It is not possible or practical to undertake an economic study alongside every
  clinical trial. In many cases, clinical trials will have already been undertaken and, therefore, cost data are applied retrospectively from other sources.
  Where relevant clinical data are not available expert opinion on likely outcomes is sought.
- Where clinical trials measure intermediate endpoints or have only a short-
  term follow-up, models are used to extrapolate beyond the trial to a final
  endpoint.
- Even when RCTs are designed to collect economic data, they often fall short
  of representing the reality of routine clinical practice, and models can be
  built to correct these problems.

The most common approach used is in the form of a decision tree where the
probabilities of different options are modelled, drawing on evidence where it
is available and expert opinion where it is not. Decision analysis is based on
the theory of expected utility.[12] Expected utility is calculated by multiplying the
probability of an outcome by its utility. By constructing a decision tree the cost
for each expected utility can be calculated (Figure 11.2).

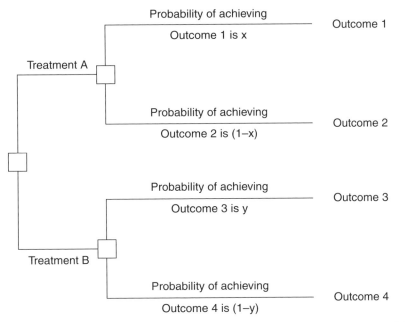

Figure 11.2:   A decision tree is an analytical framework representing choices available, outcomes and probabilities of achieving those outcomes. The choice made depends on the cost and expected value of each option. Decision trees can be used to improve decision making and illuminate the data that is required to make a decision.

Although modelling is used widely in economic analysis it has been criticised in a number of areas:[13]

- it oversimplifies reality
- assumptions are often subjective and liable to bias
- danger of 'data mining' – if enough options are considered, a result will be found
- danger of extrapolating long-term outcomes from short-term data.

Problems with economic modelling are clearly demonstrated by the report of NICE on the use of beta interferon for multiple sclerosis[14] that found model estimates of cost per QALY of between £10,000 and $3 million!

Guidelines for economic studies

Although there is a general consensus among experts on the existence of the number of basic principles governing the design of such studies, many issues

---

Box 11.4:   Questions to ask of an economic evaluation

- Was a well defined question posed in an answerable form?
- Was a comprehensive description of the competing alternatives given?
- Was there evidence that the programme's effectiveness had been established?
- Were all the important and relevant costs and consequences for each alternative identified?
- Were costs and consequences measured accurately in appropriate physical units?
- Were costs and consequences valued credibly?
- Were costs and consequences adjusted for different timing?
- Was an incremental analysis of cost and consequences of alternatives performed?
- Was a sensitivity analysis performed?
- Did a presentation and discussion of study results include all issues of concern to users?

---

remain unresolved.[15] Guidelines have been developed to maintain consistency and compatibility across economic studies,[16,17] and some countries such as Australia and Canada stipulate guidelines for formal economic analysis that any new drug must undergo before it can be introduced.

However, it has been suggested that guidelines might unnecessarily stifle methodological development and that value judgements made in economic evaluation could quite legitimately vary from setting to setting. Consequently, any efforts to standardise methodology should be developmental rather than static.[18] Others have argued that the investment in the improvement of guidelines and the development of a consensus about best practice yields only a small marginal improvement and these resources may be better invested in other areas of health economics.[19] Box 11.4 shows the basics of good practice in any economic evaluation.[20]

Conclusion

This chapter has considered some problems of collecting and analysing economic data. Although guidelines have been developed for this exercise, there remain many areas where consensus has yet to be obtained. However, even when data have been obtained they need to be assessed and acted on in a way that is accessible to end users. This aspect forms the basis of the next chapter.

References

1 Black D (1998) The limitations of evidence. *J R Coll Phys*. **32**: 23–6.
2 Hammond K (1998) Clinical intuition and clinical analysis: expertise and the cognitive continuum. In: J Dowie and A Elstein (eds) *Professional Judgment: a reader in clinical decision making*. Cambridge University Press, Cambridge.
3 Jan S (1998) A holistic approach to the economic evaluation of health programs using institutionalism methodology. *Soc Sci Med*. **47(10)**: 1565–72.
4 Byford S and Raftery J (1998) Perspectives in economic evaluation. *BMJ*. **316**: 152–9.
5 Torgerson DJ and Raftery J (1999) Economics notes: discounting. *BMJ*. **319**: 914–15.
6 Torgerson DJ and Spencer A (1996) Marginal costs and benefits. *BMJ*. **312**: 35–6.
7 Pharoah P and Hollingworth W (1996) Cost effectiveness of lowering cholesterol concentration in patients with and without pre-existing coronary heart disease: life table method applied to health authority population. *BMJ*. **312**: 1443–8.
8 O'Brian B, Drummond MF, Labell ER *et al*. (1994) In search of power and significance: issues in the design and analysis of stochastic economic appraisals. *Medical Care*. **32**: 150–63.
9 Thompson J and Barber A (2000) How should cost data in randomised trials be analysed? *BMJ*. **320**: 1197–200.
10 Sassi F, Archard I and LeGrand J (2001) Equity and economic evaluation of healthcare. *Health Technol Assess*. **5(3)**.
11 Rittenhouse B (1996) *Use of Models in Economic Evaluations of Medicines and other Healthcare Technologies*. Office of Health Economics, London.
12 Elwyn G, Edwards A, Eccles M *et al*. (2001) Decision analysis in patient care. *Lancet*. **358**: 571–4.
13 Buxton M, Drummond M, Van Hoult B, Prince R *et al*. (1997) Modelling in economic evaluation: an unavoidable fact of life. *Health Economics*. **6**: 217–27.
14 NICE (2002) *NICE Technology Appraisal Guidance No. 32*. NICE, London.
15 Hutton J (1994) Economic evaluation of healthcare: a half way technology. *Health Economics*. **3**: 1–4.
16 Drummond M (1994) Economic analysis alongside control trials. DoH, London.
17 Drummond MF and Jefferson TD (1996) Guidelines for authors and peer reviewers of economic submissions to the BMJ. *BMJ*. **313**: 275–83.
18 Drummond MF and Davies L (1991) Economic analysis alongside clinical trials: revisiting the methodological issues. *International J Technology Assess Health Care*. **7(4)**: 561–73.
19 Maynard A (1997) Economic evaluation techniques in healthcare: reinventing the wheel? *Pharmacoeconomics*. **11(2)**: 115–18.
20 Drummond M, Stoddard G and Torrance G (1987) *Methods of Economic Evaluation of Healthcare Programmes*. Oxford University Press, Oxford.

CHAPTER 12

Using information from economic evaluations

David Kernick

Health economic information needs to be collated, synthesised and appraised in such a way that it is helpful to decision makers. However, the methods for summarising and presenting the findings of economic evaluation is are not as well established as for clinical evidence. This chapter outlines how the results of economic evaluation can be presented to decision makers.

Key points

- Commissioners and practitioners have neither the time nor the expertise to collect, synthesise and analyse economic information.
- Methods of presenting economic data in a way that is helpful to decision makers are not well developed.
- Tabular summaries offer simple decision rules, but in many cases decisions may not be clear cut, and a decision has to be made whether the increase in benefit of an intervention is commensurate with the increase in its cost.
- Threshold approaches suggest a threshold monetary value for an outcome that society is willing to pay.
- Consensus panels consider inputs from a number of sources and make graded recommendations according to the strength of evidence on which they are based.

Chapter sections

- **Introduction**
- **Tabular summaries**
- **Threshold value approach**
- **Developing consensus policy guidelines**
- **Conclusion**

Introduction

Policy makers need to take into account results of healthcare experiments. In the field of clinical effectiveness, methods of synthesising data and summarising results are well advanced and statistically robust. However, the methodology for summarising the findings of economic evaluation and developing decision guidelines is not well developed.

For some types of evaluation, results are clear cut. For example, if a cost minimisation exercise is undertaken, the cheapest option will be chosen. In cost benefit analysis, if the cost savings exceed the cost of the intervention then the programme should be implemented. However, the most common types of evaluations are cost effectiveness or cost utility studies which usually do not generate a simple answer.

In some cases economic evaluations underpin decisions that are mandatory. For example, in Canada and Australia new drugs have to demonstrate they are cost effective before they can be licensed. In the UK, the emphasis is on economic evaluations informing guidelines issued under the auspices of the National Institute for Clinical Excellence (NICE) that are not mandatory although this may well change. We await with interest to see what happens if decisions become mandatory and practitioners elect not to follow the guidelines on a significant scale! The work of NICE is considered in Chapter 20 and legal aspects of this area in Chapter 23.

The simplest approach to presenting economic data is a factual summary of the results of a study, but decision makers may have neither the time nor expertise to synthesise and analyse this information. This chapter reviews the three main approaches that can be used to present economic information to decision makers.

Tabular summaries

The most elementary method of summarising the results of economic studies is in the form of a tabular display. Table 12.1 shows a permutation matrix for possible outcomes of an economic evaluation of an intervention against a comparator. Other variations around this theme have been suggested, such as a hierarchical table, but the principle is the same.[1]

If more than one study has been undertaken the number of studies can be shown in each table sector. Certain results give clear cut decisions. For example, better outcomes and lower cost are clearly accepted. Higher costs and worst outcomes would be rejected. However, in many cases there will be no clear preference – a new intervention may cost more but give more benefit. In this case, the decision has to be made as to whether the increased benefit is commensurate with the increase in cost. One approach is to present data grouped in a league table of cost effectiveness ratios – the additional cost of obtaining a

Table 12.1: Decision rules for cost effectiveness or cost utility analysis. Changes in costs and benefits of new interventions compared with comparator

Cost compared with comparator	Benefit compared with comparator	Action
Reduced	Reduced	Don't use
Reduced	Same or enhanced	Use
Increased	Same or reduced	Don't use
Increased	Increased	Is the increment in cost worth the additional benefit?

health effect from a given intervention when compared with comparator. This allows decision makers to establish a relevant opportunity cost. An example is shown in Table 12.2. However, the use of cost effectiveness league tables are not without problems,[2] some of which are shown in Box 12.1.

Table 12.2: A cost effectiveness league table. Cost per quality adjusted life year (QALY) of competing therapies – some tentative estimates[3]

Intervention	Cost per QALY (1990 prices)
GP advice to stop smoking	£270
Antihypertensive therapy	£940
Pacemaker insertion	£1100
Hip replacement	£1180
Valve replacement for aortic stenosis	£1410
Coronary artery bypass graft	£2090
Kidney transplant	£4710
Breast screening	£5780
Heart transplant	£7840
Hospital haemodialysis	£21,970

Box 12.1: Some problems with cost effectiveness league tables

- Results have a shelf life.
- Methodologies vary.
- Comparators may differ.
- Studies may not be generalisable.
- Studies have large resource implications – not every intervention can undergo economic evaluation.
- They ignore affordability. Even when an intervention is efficient, it may not be affordable if it is applicable to a large number of the population.

Threshold value approach

Other approaches have suggested a threshold value for the QALY that society is willing to pay. Table 12.3 shows one possible framework based on the quality of evidence on which the economic study is based, suggesting that interventions based on good evidence and costing up to £20,000 for each additional QALY are probably worth paying for.[4] However, this approach overlooks affordability. If a new intervention delivers QALYs under the threshold but is widely applicable, there could be uncontrollable healthcare expenditure. There is also the likelihood that manufacturers will price their products at the threshold value, again leading to budgetary pressures. There does seem to be a suggestion, albeit denied, that NICE is looking at a threshold value of around £30,000 per QALY.

Table 12.3:   A suggested framework to decide whether an intervention should be adopted based on the strength of evidence and cost/QALY

Quality of evidence	A	B	C
Strong evidence (RCT)	++	++	±
Good evidence (non-RCT)	++	+	±
Expert opinion	+	±	±
Inadequate evidence	0	0	0

A: <£3000 per life year (or QALY equivalent)
B: £3000–£20,000
C: Over £20,000

Developing consensus policy guidelines

Clinical and economic evidence about the benefit and harm of interventions is often incomplete, and techniques for analysing and projecting costs and benefits are complex and still evolving. Policy makers also need to accommodate other inputs, which include affordability, equity and consumer input. There is rarely a simple yes or no answer to any resource allocation decision.

One approach is to convene a panel of relevant stakeholders who formulate treatment recommendations. The workings of the group can be characterised as a dynamic process in which an understanding of the pros and cons of treatment emerges and uncertainties are assessed.[5] There are a number of factors contributing to this process which include:

- the nature of the evidence
- the generalisability of the evidence

- resource implications of the process itself
- knowledge of the healthcare system
- beliefs and values of the panel
- political directives.

A major problem with guideline development is that it requires considerable investment in resources and its recommendations can go out of date quite quickly. New studies are being continually published and costs on which economic evaluations are based can change.

The area has been reviewed extensively by Eccles[6] (www.ncchta.org) who emphasises a number of points.

- It is important to be clear about the process and objective of guideline development, the conduct of meetings and the role of each group member.
- A guideline group should contain a number of professionals including health economists, statisticians, epidemiologists and health service researchers.
- Important inputs to a decision-making process include effectiveness, side effects, compliance, safety, quality of life, health service delivery issues, resource use and costs.
- The outcomes of the guideline process are usually graded treatment recommendations that reflect some or all of the above attributes.
- Where it is appropriate, uncertainty should be explored.
- The importance attached to each attribute of treatment remains the responsibility of the guideline development group, but must be transparent and credible to the target audience. When modelling studies are used, they should be simple and transparent to allow exploration with the application of different values.
- Guideline panels should not be afraid to say, 'we just don't know yet and further research is required'.

Box 12.2 shows an example of a consensus guideline that incorporates economic data.

Box 12.2:   An example of a consensus guideline that incorporates economic data. Guidelines developed by a development group considering the treatment of depression in primary care with tricyclic antidepressants (TCAs) or serotonin selective reuptake inhibitor drugs (SSRIs)[7]

- TCAs are the most cost effective option for the treatment of depression and should be used as routine first-line treatment in primary care.
- The ultimate choice of antidepressant should be based on patient factors which would include:

- desirability or otherwise of sedation
- previous response to a particular drug
- comorbid, psychiatric or medical conditions
- concurrent drug therapy.

- If the toxic effects of the older TCAs are perceived to be a problem in patients who have previously taken an overdose or the elderly, then Lofepramine is a more cost effective choice than an SSRI.

Conclusion

This chapter has considered some problems of analysing and presenting economic data and putting the results of studies into action. Economic evaluation offers a useful framework that can facilitate the difficult choices with which decision makers are confronted and ensure that resources are used in an efficient manner. However, to date, the impact of economic evaluation on decisions at all levels of healthcare has been limited. One reason may be because decision makers have not been given information in a way that is accessible, understandable and relevant to their circumstances. There has been no widely accepted way of incorporating economic considerations into practice. In view of the complex inputs into any resource decision, it may be that the development of consensus policy guidelines may offer the best way forward.

References

1 Nixon J, Carn K and Kleijnen J (2001) Summarising economic evaluations in systematic reviews: a new approach. *BMJ.* **322:** 1596–8.
2 Gerard K and Mooney G (1993) QALY league tables – handle with care. *Health Economics.* **2:** 59–64.
3 Drummond M and Maynard A (1993) *Purchasing and Providing Cost Effective Healthcare.* Churchill Livingstone, London.
4 Stevens A, Colin-Jones D and Gabbay J (1995) Quick and clean: authoritative health technology assessment for local healthcare contracting. *Health Trends.* **37:** 37–42.
5 Eccles M, Freemantle N and Mason J (1998) North of England evidence-based guidelines development project: methods of developing guidelines for efficient drug use in primary care. *BMJ.* **316:** 1232–5.
6 Eccles M and Mason J (2001) How to develop cost conscious guidelines. *Health Technol Assess.* **5(16).**
7 Eccles M, Freemantle N and Mason J (1999) North of England evidence based guidelines development project: summary version of guidelines for the choice of antidepressants for depression in primary care. *Fam Pract.* **16:** 103–11.

Section 4

Getting economic evaluation into practice

Health economic theory will be of little use if it is not adopted and used in practice. This section considers how decision makers can use the results of economic evaluation. Economic studies on medicines have formed the core of economic evaluations and will be the area with which most practitioners are familiar. However, pharmacoeconomics is characterised by a number of specific issues that Tom Walley explores in Chapter 13.

Against a background of government calls for a radical change in the way in which the medical workforce is planned and trained, the concept of skill mix seeks to match clinical presentation to an intervention based on an appropriate level of skill and training. However, unless the economic issues are thought through clearly, there is a danger that resources may be utilised inefficiently. In Chapter 14, Anthony Scott and I outline the economic issues in this area and offer a pragmatic framework that can facilitate skill mix decisions.

The continuing emphasis on a primary care led NHS has seen a shift of services from secondary to primary care ahead of an evidence base of both effectiveness and cost effectiveness. In Chapter 15, we outline some of the problems encountered from an economic perspective when shifting services across the secondary/primary care interface and highlight barriers to progress in this area. We conclude that attention should be focused on improving efficiency at the interface through cooperation and communication, rather than shifting services across it.

The most rapidly growing sector of healthcare is the field of complementary and alternative medicine. In the USA, more people are visiting complementary therapists than doctors. In Chapter 16, Adrian White and I review the difficulties of obtaining economic data in this area, but suggest that the subject may open a broader agenda about the meaning of health and the benefits that we should be looking for in an economic study.

The last decade has seen an exponential rise in the publication of cost effectiveness studies. In Chapter 17, Ruth McDonald and I argue that the volume of economic evaluations produced have not been commensurate with their impact on policy making at grassroots level and explore why this might be. Ruth goes on to explore programme budgeting and marginal analysis in Chapter 18, arguably the most pragmatic approach to economic evaluation. She finds that despite its practical appeal, it has yet to find widespread implementation in practice.

CHAPTER 13

Pharmacoeconomics

Tom Walley

The current drugs bill in the NHS is now over £5 billion a year. The ease with which this spending can be identified has focused attention on medicines as an important approach to reducing costs, and the move towards single unified budgets in primary care offers a way to ensure a more efficient utilisation of spending in this area. However, the application of health economics to pharmaceuticals is compounded by a number of specific issues. These relate to the need for government to control costs while achieving maximum value for money, the difficulty of establishing a relevant and unbiased evidence base of cost effectiveness and the need to support an important sector of British industry.

Key points
- Pharmacoeconomics is the application of health economics to medicines and draws on the same techniques.
- The high cost of medicines and the ease of identifying these costs encourage attention on drug costs rather than cost effectiveness.
- Medicines are easier to evaluate economically than many other medical interventions because of the high quality of information required for licensing.
- Economic evaluation of medicines is essential if we are to focus on the value of medicines rather than their costs.
- Such evaluations may be misused as marketing or as a means of controlling government spending.

Chapter sections
- **Introduction**
- **The costs of medicines**
- **Providing evidence to support pharmaceutical interventions**
- **The commercial influences on economic studies and their use in marketing**
- **The use of pharmacoeconomics by government**
- **Conclusion**

Introduction

Spending on medicines is a target for savings in healthcare costs for governments around the world. This comes about because of the size of the medicine bill (over £5 billion in the UK), because pharmaceutical costs are easily measured, and finally because there is thought to be waste in prescribing. Government attempts to contain the medicine bill around the world include increased patient copayments, prescribing lists or formularies, and indicative or real medicine budgets.[1] This focuses on simple medicine costs, however, when what should be of greater concern to us all is the value of medicines – a function of their benefits as well as their costs.[2] After all, it is not the function of a health service to save money, but to use its limited resources to achieve the greatest health gain for its population. By these criteria, spending on medicines, which may for instance reduce the need for hospitalisation or produce greater health gain for the same resources than other interventions, may be highly efficient. Medicine costs should, therefore, not be considered in isolation from other healthcare costs. This assessment of the costs and benefits is difficult, but essential for a health service determined to use its resources most wisely.

The role of health economics is to undertake this assessment – not to save money, but to make explicit the use of resources and the consequences of alternative use of resources, so as to inform our decisions. The term 'pharmacoeconomics' refers to the application of health economics to pharmaceuticals. Many health economists dislike the term, arguing that there is nothing unique about pharmaceuticals, or the application of health economics to them. Of course this argument is correct, but nevertheless there are specific issues around the application of health economics to pharmaceuticals. The key issues are:

- the costs of medicines and the identification of these costs
- the evidence behind pharmacoeconomic evaluations and how that evidence is obtained
- the commercial influences on the studies and their use in marketing
- the use of pharmacoeconomics by agencies such as the National Institute for Clinical Excellence (NICE) in the UK or similar agencies elsewhere.

The costs of medicines

The cost of medicines in the NHS and other health services around the world is substantial and rising. In the UK, drugs consume about 12% of total NHS costs, the second biggest element after salaries. Figure 13.1 shows that drug costs have almost doubled in the last 10 years. About 80% of all prescribing costs are spent

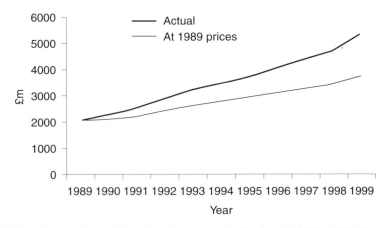

Figure 13.1:   Costs of prescribing in primary care in England, 1989–1999 (Department of Health, 2000).

in primary care. While it is artificial to separate out the costs of medicines from the costs of the whole management of the patient, medicine costs are easily identifiable to the last penny, and are fed back to GPs as PACT (Prescribing Analysis and CosT) data. It is, in part, the ease with which this spending can be identified and its separation from other aspects of care which has focused so much attention on the medicine bill in recent years. This is in contrast to other areas of healthcare, such as surgical procedures or hospital admissions, for which the costs in the NHS are often difficult to define.

This is not to discount the importance of knowing what a medicine costs, of which prescribers are generally ignorant,[3] nor to discount which medicine is most effective and safe for a given indication. Where two medicines are equal in effectiveness and safety, it is irresponsible to spend money unnecessarily on the more expensive. This is the justification for generic prescribing which is usually less expensive than prescribing branded medicines. However, for too long the discussion around medicine costs has been limited to costs alone, and has often been aimed at cost containment rather than also considering the benefits.

The move towards unified budgets

For many years, prescribing budgets were the fashion but these have now been subsumed into the single unified budgets of primary care groups or trusts in England. This seems a more reasonable way to examine the costs of managing the patient (e.g. in the dyspeptic patient, the decision on whether to perform endoscopy is of more consequence than the choice of a proton pump inhibitor medication).

The single unified budget has a further advantage in pharmacoeconomics. An expensive medicine may impact on the prescribing budget, but might make savings elsewhere in the NHS, for instance by reducing hospital admissions. These savings were not in any budget that the prescriber had access to and so were less directly relevant to the prescriber. With the unified budget such savings should now be real (provided the contracting process can be made to work). Conversely, the opportunity costs of high medicine spending in terms of reduction of other services were often invisible to the prescriber but now are much clearer.

The pricing of drugs

In many countries, there are schemes whereby the prices of medicines are regulated by government. In the UK, however, there is a unique system not of regulating medicine prices but of regulating the profits of the industry. This is achieved by means of a scheme negotiated between government and the pharmaceutical industry – the Pharmaceutical Pricing Regulatory Scheme (PPRS).[4] Under this, companies are allowed to make profits from their NHS sales in accordance with the amount of capital they have invested in the UK. Typical permitted profits are of the order of 10–12%, a handsome return.

The PPRS has two aims, the first of which is to secure reasonable prices for the NHS. Any company overspending its 'target' profit has to return money to the Treasury, and companies adjust their prices so as not to exceed this. The second is to promote the British pharmaceutical industry and encourage investment, and in this the PPRS seems very successful. Clearly, there are tensions between these two aims. Some argue that any attempt to contain medicine spending is undermined because if a company does not achieve its target profit, it may be allowed price rises in order to regain the target level. The PPRS seems contrary to several other government initiatives such as NICE (see below) and attempts to control the medicines bill.

Providing evidence to support pharmaceutical interventions

Public regulation

Medicines are carefully regulated largely for issues of public health and safety. After the thalidomide disaster of the early 1960s, most countries in the world set up systems to evaluate the safety (in particular) and the efficacy of new medicines. In the UK, these functions are served by an independent expert committee, the Committee on Safety of Medicines (CSM), supported by the Medicines Control Agency. The European Medicines Evaluation Agency is also of increasing importance. Under the Medicines Act (1968), the CSM considers the efficacy of a new medicine (i.e. can it do what it is supposed to?), its safety (is it as least as safe as other medicines for the same purpose on the market?), and whether it is manufactured to a high quality. Note that, by law, it may not consider whether a medicine is even as effective as an existing medicine, the need for a medicine, the cost of a medicine, nor its cost effectiveness. Why is the remit so limited? The answer lies in the aim of the law to promote medicine safety, while not constraining the pharmaceutical industry's profitability or innovativeness.

The regulatory agencies lay down clear criteria for evaluating the efficacy and safety of medicines involving *in vitro* and animal studies, as well as defining the terms of human exposure. The key instrument for the evaluation of the medicine in humans is the controlled clinical trial. The design and conduct of such studies are very well established, and studies have to be of the highest quality to pass the rigorous review of the regulators. Once the regulators are satisfied, they issue a licence to the manufacturer who can then sell the medicine.

An effect of this is that when we come to examine the economic implications of a medicine, there exists a wealth of extremely high quality data on its efficacy, before the medicine has even been prescribed openly. Contrast this to the average surgical or policy intervention where there is often very little good evidence. Pharmaceuticals are, therefore, more easily evaluated than many other interventions.

Problems using regulatory evidence for economic evaluation

However, there are problems with using this evidence for economic evaluations; many trials do not reflect the real world management of a condition in a particular country, but are artificially constrained so as to meet the needs of the regulatory agencies and the all-important licence. Clinical trials do not identify what is really essential for an economic evaluation of a medicine. In the clinical trial, for example, patients are highly selected and monitored, while in everyday practice patient selection is less well defined, monitoring is less rigorous and other issues such as patient compliance with therapy have an effect. Clinical trials will also fail to take into account other important issues, and often compare one medicine to another (or even to placebo) instead of, say, one line of management with another (e.g. the differences between omeprazole and lansoprazole are trivial compared to the bigger question of what is the most effective and cost effective way to manage dyspepsia).

Despite these limitations, there is a body of evidence which lends itself to economic evaluation at a very early stage of a medicine's life, which simply does not exist for other interventions.[2] Ways around this include 'naturalistic' or 'pragmatic' trials, usually conducted once the medicine is licensed and marketed, in which routine patients are prescribed the medicine or its alternative, and then followed to examine the benefits they experience in practice, and the costs (e.g. time off work, visits to GP etc). These trials are time consuming and expensive, but provide extensive useful pharmacoeconomic data and allow for a better assessment of the true value and cost of a medicine. Other ways to address the information gap between clinical trial and common practice are to use a group of expert advisers, or to perform mathematical modelling on how a different pattern of care might affect the costs and benefits. These approaches are much less satisfactory but more common than the pragmatic trial, simply because of the time and expense involved.

The commercial influences on economic studies and their use in marketing

Pharmaceutical companies have often invested £200–£300 million in developing an important new medicine, and require a return on this investment. They will, therefore, try their utmost to sell their product, recoup the investment and make further profits (which will also help fund the development of new medicines in the future). Although this exercise may be criticised in a number of areas we have to accept that we live in a free market economy directed by the profit motive.

However, new medicines rarely if ever cost less than the medicine they might replace. Companies face an increasingly uphill struggle to sell their products; the purchasers no longer buy a new medicine (as was often the case in the past) just because it is new and therefore presumably better, irrespective of cost. Purchasers and prescribers now demand evidence of the superiority over existing medicines and of the value of that superiority. Companies, therefore, have to produce economic evaluations of their products in order to convince their customers. They will argue that a new more expensive medicine is worth the extra cost because of the extra benefits it brings (e.g. clinical benefits such as more patients cured or improved, or economic benefits such as fewer hospital admissions etc.). In contrast to the controlled clinical trial, however, there is no regulatory body that supervises and reviews economic evaluations. Such evaluations are often undertaken within companies not by the highly scientific research divisions, but by the marketing divisions. These have an ethos driven not to producing a safe and effective medicine but to selling. The company studies often tend to favour their product more than an evaluation conducted by independent bodies might – easily achieved, for instance, by using favourable assumptions, selecting which costs to include and which to exclude and so on. A health economist might be aware of these issues in reading an economic evaluation of a medicine, but marketing is aimed at doctors without such training. Many economic evaluations conducted by or funded by companies are best seen as marketing activity, and have in the past given economic evaluation of medicines a bad name.[5] Prescribers need to be aware of this potential bias in such studies – caveat emptor!

The use of pharmacoeconomics by government

A large part of the rising costs of medicines is due to new medicines displacing old, which may or may not be appropriate. Most countries are developing mechanisms to evaluate new innovative technologies (including medicines) to decide whether they should be used in a health service and if so how. For instance, it may be that a new medicine is licensed for its efficacy, safety and quality of manufacture (three hurdles), but is twice as expensive as an existing medicine with the same properties. Such a drug may be legally prescribed, but a health service needs to take a view on whether it should be used. An economic evaluation to define value for money is vital in this, and is for the industry a 'fourth hurdle'. There is a good case for keeping such considerations separate from the medicine licensing process – if it were not, might we license a not-very-safe medicine because it was extremely cheap?

The UK experience

Some countries or regions have set up very formal and rigid systems to determine which medicines should be reimbursed by the state. In the UK, the relevant agency is NICE[6] which has the role of not just evaluating medicines but of other new technologies as well. So far, however, about two-thirds of its work has been medicine related. It reviews new medicines both clinically and economically and then presents 'guidance' on which, managerially if not legally, is taken to be the NHS standard of practice.

The advice NICE has provided so far has in some instances been controversial. With regard to medicines, it seems so far that no decisions based solely on the economic evaluation have been made but most are clinically based. Many decisions seem to do nothing more than rubber stamp the terms of the medicine licence. Initially, NICE was a source of great concern to the pharmaceutical industry who saw it as a potential major barrier to access to the UK market. In practice, it has not so far taken this role and many managers and professionals in the NHS have expressed disquiet[7] that NICE has, as they see it, failed to control the tide of new medicines, many of uncertain value. Even worse, NICE in its decisions has made some treatments a standard when the NHS has inadequate resources to deliver the treatment (e.g. taxanes, glycoprotein IIb/IIIa receptor antagonists) – rating effectiveness perhaps over affordability and not considering the consequences and opportunity costs of some of its decisions. This undermines local decision making and priorities, and reduces confidence in NICE. This would be unfortunate as the role of NICE is clearly vital to the NHS. The work of NICE is discussed in more length in Chapter 20.

The international experience

Pharmacoeconomic evaluation is standard practice in Australia before a new medicine will be reimbursed within the Pharmaceutical Benefits Scheme, and both doctors and patients have reported relatively few difficulties in working within the limited formulary available to them as a result. Similarly, the province of Ontario in Canada has been rigorous in evaluating new medicines and approving them for reimbursement by the provincial health service.[8] Within the USA, individual purchasers such as health maintenance organisations or government agencies similarly operate limited formularies, based in part on pharmacoeconomic evaluations. In practice, such efforts have only partly restrained the rising costs of prescribing as the new clinically valuable medicines are the main drivers and few countries have the political will to deny these to patients.

A key factor in Australia has been the lack of an innovative pharmaceutical industry, and therefore the Australians can buy their medicines as cheaply as possible on the international market without needing to consider supporting a major employer or exporter. Nor are they worried about paying for the development of innovative medicines in the future. For European countries with national health services of some kind and with large pharmaceutical industries, the willingness to restrain costs may be tempered by concerns about maintaining industry and employment. Many European countries have set up agencies similar to NICE but none have so far been as active; many seem to be waiting to learn from the British experience.

Conclusion

Pharmacoeconomics is no more than the application of health economics to pharmaceuticals. There are some specific issues around this, however, relating to the established means of evaluating medicines, the powerful commercial sponsors and the desires of government to control medicine costs while achieving maximum value for money. The structures of the health service also play a vital role in this. In one form or another, pharmacoeconomics will be of great importance to manufacturers, prescribers, administrators and patients in the foreseeable future.

References

1   Walley T, Barton S and Haycox A (1977) Drug rationing in the UK NHS: current status and future prospects. *Pharmacoeconomics.* **12:** 339–50.
2   Walley T (1995) Medicines, money and society. *Br J Clin Pharmacol.* **39:** 343–5.
3   Ryan M, Yule B, Bond C and Taylor R (1996) Do physicians' perceptions of drug costs influence their prescribing? *Pharmacoeconomics.* **9:** 321–31.
4   Earl-Slater A (1997) Regulating the price of the UK's drugs: second thoughts after the government's first report. *BMJ.* **314:** 365.
5   Drummond MF (1992) Economic evaluation of pharmaceuticals: marketing or science? *Pharmacoeconomics.* **1:** 8–13.
6   Rawlins M (1999) In pursuit of quality: the National Institute for Clinical Excellence. *Lancet.* **353:** 1079–82.
7   Smith R (2000) The failings of NICE. *BMJ.* **321:** 1363–4.
8   Freemantle N, Henry D, Maynard A and Torrance G (1995) Promoting cost effective prescribing. *BMJ.* **310:** 955–6.

CHAPTER 14

Economic evaluation and doctor/nurse skill mix

David Kernick and Anthony Scott

Against a background of government calls for a radical change in the way the medical workforce is planned and trained, the concept of skill mix seeks to match clinical presentation to an intervention based on an appropriate level of skill and training. Health economics is not the only framework within which these changes can be analysed. However, unless the economic issues are thought through clearly there is a danger that resources may be utilised inefficiently.

The aims of this chapter are to outline the economic issues in the area of doctor/nurse skill mix and concludes by offering a pragmatic framework that can facilitate decisions in this area. Although this paper is written from the perspective of primary care, it is equally relevant to skill mix in the secondary care sector.

Key points
- There has been an unplanned three-fold expansion of nurses in primary care over the past 10 years.
- It has been suggested that between 30–70% of tasks performed by doctors could be carried out satisfactorily by nurses.
- At a time of increasing demands on limited resources, the development of skill mix is an attractive proposition for policy makers.
- The allocation of skill mix should be directed by considerations of effectiveness, resource use and patient satisfaction.
- There are a number of problems obtaining clinical and economic evidence in this area.

Chapter sections
- **Introduction**
- **Using economic evaluation to facilitate skill mix choices**

> - A pragmatic framework that can facilitate skill mix decisions from an economic perspective
> - Conclusion

Introduction

The current healthcare environment is characterised by rapid change, financial constraint, a shift in professional boundaries and more complex healthcare needs. Nearly one million people work for the NHS and these factors have prompted the search for new ways of configuring the healthcare workforce that improves the efficient and equitable delivery of care.

A recent government review of the way in which the NHS educates, trains and uses its staff outlined a range of wide ranging and radical proposals.[1] The review recognises that current workforce planning and development arrangements inhibit the development of multiprofessional planning and have not supported the creative use of staff skills. It stressed the need for greater integration of workforce planning and development, with service and financial planning combined with more flexible deployment of staff to maximise the use of their skills and abilities.

A number of proposals are made to achieve these ends that include:

- workforce planning and development to be aligned with service planning at local level through the Health Improvement Programme (HImP)
- workforce plans to be developed on a multidisciplinary basis, focusing on services to be delivered and looking across primary, secondary and tertiary care
- the establishment of a national workforce development board, supported by care group workforce development boards, to be responsible for ensuring the proper integration of workforce issues, with service development taking account of skill mix changes and research and development findings
- central action to coordinate work on skill mix changes and the development of new types of healthcare worker.

Box 14.1 shows some current pressures to reconfigure the doctor/nurse workforce.

In the last 10 years, the number of nurses employed in general practice has trebled and it has been estimated that there are now 94,000 whole time equivalents working in primary care. Practice nurses are advising on acute problems, participate in clinics for chronic disease and provide health education and counselling.[2] This expansion had not been centrally planned but evolved from

Box 14.1:   Pressures influencing the reconfiguration of the doctor/nurse workforce

- The workforce is a major expenditure of the NHS budget. Against a background of increasing demands on limited resources, there is a need to ensure efficient utilisation of this workforce.
- A more educated nursing sector has resulted in pressure on existing professional boundaries and access to many areas that were previously the prerogative of doctors.
- An evidence base is developing which suggests that in many clinical areas, roles undertaken by doctors can be successfully transferred to nurses. Nurse led personal medical services pilots have demonstrated that nurses can also lead the delivery of primary care.[2]
- An emphasis on a more holistic approach to care and a focus on prevention and health promotion has been claimed to be better suited to the characteristics of nursing.

the 1990 GP contract. GPs were encouraged to provide screening and health promotion services and did so by delegating these roles to their practice nurses.

In a literature review, Richardson and Maynard[4] suggested that 30–70% of tasks performed by doctors could be carried out satisfactorily by nurses. This had significant implications for medical manpower but most studies were undertaken in North America where nurses have established a leading role in the provision of primary medical care. Although the concept of team working has been accepted throughout the NHS,[5] there still remains limited evidence of effectiveness and virtually none of cost effectiveness to justify current practice or base the expansion of the practice nurse role within primary care.

Working in teams

The concept of skill mix seeks to match clinical presentations with an intervention based on an appropriate level of skill and training.[6] Working in teams allows health professionals to contribute their unique assets towards the attainment of a common goal, and a commitment to a primary care led NHS based on teamwork has added urgency to the debate (Table 14.1). Evidence to support the traditional doctor centred model of care where the GP provides medical continuity has not been forthcoming and over the past decade there has been a shift in emphasis towards a multidisciplinary team approach which has the

Table 14.1:   Some advantages and disadvantages of working in teams[8]

Advantages of teamworking	Disadvantages of teamworking
• Diffusion of information and learning • Mutual monitoring • Group cohesion • Risk pooling (sharing impact of beneficial and adverse events) • Economies of scale • Division of labour	• Team members may reduce effort if monitoring of effort is difficult, while benefiting from the effort of others ('free riding') • Professional role and value conflict due to unequal status and power

flexibility to respond to rapidly changing health needs and in which the nurse generalist is seen as a core member.

Three types of relationship within a team have been defined.[7]

- Coactive – this relationship implies a delegation of activity and implies that one member of the relationship is in a dominant position and can identify what is delegated. Delegation remains the dominant model within primary care.
- Competitive – in this relationship, parties are not working together towards a common goal but competing for similar roles. This model is prevalent in the USA where nurses find themselves competing with doctors over prescribing and hospital admitting rights.
- Interactive – this approach implies sharing of responsibilities and a collaboration based on equality. In this interdisciplinary model, although each practitioner offers a set of individual skills professional boundaries are not well defined.

A recent report by the British Medical Association has suggested that the emphasis should be on continuity within the primary healthcare team, not that of an individual practitioner,[9] and there is a recognition of the importance of delivering health from a primary care system with the emphasis on personal responsibility, patient participation and coactive teamwork. However, how nurses and doctors can most effectively work together in primary care teams remains uncertain.

From an economics perspective, it is important to ask what types of incentives are present to encourage individuals to work in teams. The group practice allowance in the GP contract was a major force in encouraging GPs to work together in group practice until its abolition in 1991. Team-based rewards were also suggested in the recent NHS Plan. Rewarding groups rather than individuals directly links the efforts of individuals to the group reward, and may enhance cooperation and mutual monitoring depending on how group rewards are shared among members of the team.[8] Increased teamwork may help to clarify the roles, responsibilities and complementarity of team members, which may in turn lead to changes in skill mix.

Models of nurse intervention – stereotypes based on historical precedent?

The context in which a nurse intervention is to be considered is the first step in any analysis. A recent document from the Royal College of General Practitioners defined the elements of effective and efficient primary care as its accessible front line position, its longitudinal nature, its focus on the individual, its responsibility for dealing with common problems, its coordination function for integrated patient care and its orientation to prevention in addition to traditional clinical functions.[10] The consultation remains the central focus for resource allocation in primary care, and consists of identifying and prioritising the needs of the patients, negotiating with the patient resources that meet those needs and improving patients' understanding and their ability to cope with their problems. Needs are often identified and met over a series of interactions. Do nurses respond to these elements in a way that is different from doctors and that can provide better outcomes in some cases? Or do they simply represent a cheaper alternative?

In 1986, the Cumberledge Report[11] recommended the introduction of the nurse practitioner into primary care, suggesting that patients should be able to choose between consulting with a doctor or a nurse. Suitable roles were identified as securing compliance with therapy, making initial assessment of patients, and diagnosing and treating minor acute illness. Other more emotive opinions have been proffered. For example, Casey and Smith[12] saw nursing emerging as a scientific discipline that is distinct from, but complementary to medicine, emphasising the dangers of treating nurses as 'mini-doctors' and the enormous benefits that 'only nurses can offer'.

In fact, the last 20 years have seen an erosion of the nurse as an empathetic practitioner supporting patients through their daily activities and basic needs. Changes in medical practice and an emphasis on a more independent and autonomous patient have led to a new perspective for nursing care. It is difficult to differentiate the Chief Nursing Officer's 'ten key roles for nurses'[13] from key doctor roles. Despite resistance from the Royal Colleges, partnership and flexibility are becoming the key themes within a spectrum of care characterised by complexity and uncertainty, and not by unique roles that infer that nurses are different from doctors.

Management and planning treatment on the basis of the interpretation and integration of complex clinical, psychological, social, cultural and cost factors, combined with personal experience and knowledge of patients. Organising and coordinating a multidisciplinary team.	Clinical diagnosis and treatment of less complex presentations. Some areas of chronic care. Interaction with other members of the primary healthcare team.	Well-defined protocol directing clinical care in specific areas (e.g. asthma, HRT, contraception management).	Traditional nursing care (e.g. immunisation, ulcer management, management of minor injuries).	Simple, well defined task that can be undertaken with limited training (e.g. venepuncture, urine analysis, simple dressings).
Area A (GP)	Area B (nurse practitioner)	Area C (extended role practice nurse)	Area D (practice nurse)	Area E (practice nurse auxiliary)

+ .... Complexity/uncertainty of task .... −
+ .... Resource allocation/unit time .... −

Figure 14.1:   The range of tasks in primary care.

Figure 14.1 shows the range of interventions that are delivered in primary care by existing roles. Nurses and doctors are not seen to be complementary but form part of a continuum of care that seeks to optimise health gain from an appropriate use of skills and time of each practitioner. Nurses receive less training, accept less responsibility and deal with less uncertainty. As a result they receive less remuneration.

Using economic evaluation to facilitate skill mix choices

The principles of economic evaluation

An economic evaluation facilitates choice between alternative interventions by relating the health outputs (benefits) of an intervention to the resources that are consumed (Figure 14.2).[14] This exercise seeks to facilitate the efficient use of resources either by ensuring the maximum output for a given level of resource input or minimum cost to obtain a desired level of benefit (technical efficiency). It can also facilitate the most efficient mix of services provided (allocative efficiency). Inefficiency means that benefits to patients are not being

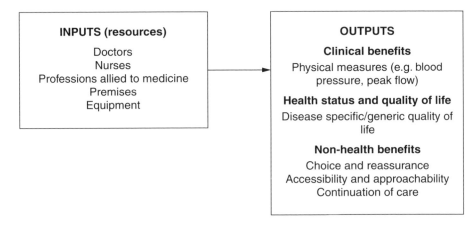

| INPUTS (resources) | OUTPUTS |

Figure 14.2:   An economic analysis relates inputs (resources) to outputs (benefits and the values attached to them) of alternative interventions to facilitate decision making when resources are scarce.

maximised, as resources are not deployed in their best use. Skill mix issues are concerned with the most efficient mix of inputs (i.e. doctors or nurses) to achieve a specific output.

For a given health condition, undertaking an economic analysis seeks to optimise skill mix accordingly within the rational framework of decision making. The steps are:

- specify the objective
- identify all relevant options for achieving the objective
- calculate the costs and benefits for each option
- choose the option which will maximise the objectives given the available resources.

However, this task is not straightforward and there are problems in all these stages.

Lack of clarity about skill mix objectives

The overall objectives of altering skill mix can be couched in terms of maintaining or improving benefits to patients, and maintaining or reducing the cost of labour. Motivations for skill mix changes in primary care usually come from the perspective of releasing the time of doctors to undertake more beneficial activities suitable to their skills. That is, nurses can substitute for doctors releasing doctor time to enhance care in other areas. For example, nurses can manage minor illness in primary care with similar outcomes to GPs.[15] Nurses have also been shown to be capable of delivering a more extensive package of primary care from nurse led primary care sites.[2] Alternatively, through substitution, medical manpower requirements can be reduced. In the former case, costs would increase as doctors' time commitment will be the same, but extra nurses will be required. In the latter case, nurse substitution would result in reduced employment for doctors. Alternatively, nurses can complement doctors, enhancing interventions in specific areas. For example, a dermatology nurse working alongside GPs can enhance the dermatology care of patients in general practice.[16] This is likely to lead to increased benefits to patients and increased costs.

A third option is that increased nurse availability may lead to additional consultations through identifying unmet need. Patients who would not have previously consulted may now do so, and there is some indirect evidence to support this. For example, a study on the impact of nurse practitioners in primary care showed no reduction in the rate of GP consultation.[10] Transfer of the management of self limiting conditions from general practice to community pharmacies showed no change in overall GP workload.[17]

Measuring costs

Many studies provide misleading conclusions for decision makers due to inappropriate cost estimates.[18] For example, a recent review of studies that derived the cost of a GP consultation found a range of between £3 and £11 depending on the method of costing used.[19] How costs are derived and combined will depend on the assumptions that have been made in their derivation and there are a number of costing rules that must be used when estimating cost data (*see* Chapter 9).

The perspective of an exercise will determine which costs to count. For example, for long-term shifts in skill mix within the NHS, training costs must be identified and allocated to the unit costs of practitioners. The annuitised costs arising from professional training are rarely considered, but will increase the cost of a GP consultation substantially (Table 14.2).

Table 14.2:   The importance of perspective. What does a GP cost? Different perspectives give different answers

What does a GP cost?[20]	
Perspective	*Cost*
GP practice	£21/hour
Health Authority (includes central overheads)	£53/hour
NHS (includes training costs)	£69/hour

Once the perspective has determined which costs to count, the concept of opportunity cost will determine how to value them. Opportunity cost is defined as the benefit foregone from using resources one way rather than another. The cost of a GP or nurse consultation may, therefore, vary depending on the value of the foregone alternative and what the GP or nurse would have otherwise been doing. Different contexts of examining skill mix may, therefore, lead to different opportunity costs. Although there still remain a number of deficiencies in cost data, estimates are becoming more accurate. A range of costs of health professionals updated annually can be found in Netten *et al.*[20]

Measuring the outcomes of skill mix options

Although health outcome measurement recognises the broader concepts of health, other sources of benefit that may be of particular relevance for nurse interventions can be overlooked.[21] For example benefit may be obtained from the process of care arising from information reassurance or choice. The relationship between structural and process variables to final health outcomes may also be tenuous in this area. Outcomes are often multidimensional and assessment may be affected by timing and characterised by difficulties with attribution.[22,23]

Ideally, all outputs should be integrated into one overall index of benefit. This is important when comparing different interventions but is rarely possible. In practice what gets measured will depend on the context of the exercise and the agency that sets the evaluation agenda. One option known as a cost consequence analysis[24] is to present outcomes in a disaggregated form allowing decision makers to make the necessary value judgements and trade-offs (*see* Chapter 11).

Relating costs to benefits

Ideally, an economic analysis should be carried out alongside a controlled trial. Where direct substitution takes place the methodology can be relatively straight forward. For example, one study randomised patients to conventional care or care exclusively from a nurse practitioner and found similar outcomes.[25] However, in most cases there will be elements of both substitution, enhancement and addition, and exact roles may be difficult to define.

In practice, most decisions will not be whether services should be totally delegated but whether resources should be shifted between existing services. A marginal analysis[26] recognises the importance of how benefits and costs change as programmes expand or contract. For example, an asthma nurse rarely provides exclusive respiratory care but shares this role with the GP, and the extent of this sharing may differ. In principle, this relationship should be determined by undertaking trials across a number of skill mix options to identify the optimum doctor/nurse mix, but this will rarely be possible.

Due to the wide variation in case-mix, training and organisation, there will inevitably be problems with generalisability, and estimates of the potential for doctor/nurse delegation may be sensitive to the methods of data collection and type of practice. Trials themselves have an opportunity cost and multicentre studies are difficult and expensive to manage especially in primary care. In summary, there will difficulties in obtaining rigorous, generalisable evidence, particularly where there are elements of both substitution and complementation.

A pragmatic framework that can facilitate skill mix decisions from an economic perspective

We have demonstrated some issues in undertaking an economic analysis in the area of doctor/nurse skill mix, particularly in primary care. Although the use of an economic framework can help clarify decision making, an exact solution to skill mix will rarely be accessible. Here, we offer a pragmatic framework that incorporates a number of economic principles that can facilitate decision making in this area.

- Identify the strategic aims of skill mix. For example, is the aim to release resources by doctor substitution for use elsewhere or to maximise health gain from additional resources by complementing the intervention of doctors?
- Identify the perspective of the exercise (i.e. who is asking the question and why?). This will determine which costs to count. For example, for long-term changes in skill mix across the NHS, training costs will be relevant.
- What are doctors and nurses currently doing in specific clinical areas, and how can this be altered to either reduce costs for the same outcome, or enhance outcomes for the same costs? This should help generate a range of skill mix options. There may be a wide range of skill mix options across which testing may not be feasible. In practice, the option considered will have to be made based on the best available evidence and expert opinion.
- What is the scope for change? It will be of little benefit to consider large scale doctor replacement if the required number of nurses are not available, or to reduce GPs in a practice if no one is retiring. Often, there will be limited room for manoeuvre in the short term. Change may only be possible over longer periods if suitable incentives and policies are in place.

- What are the likely changes in costs and benefits of each skill mix option, compared to the current allocation of tasks and time? The evidence base may be limited and not easy to generalise, and often the opinions and experiences of local commissioners and providers of care will be relevant.

Conclusion

The development of skill mix is a complex area that can be approached using a number of different analytical frameworks. For example Pratt et al.[27] emphasise the importance of exploring purpose and building relationships, and argue that coevolution of partners is the most relevant mode building on the strengths of each partner. Senge[28] sees teams as part of a learning organisation where team learning exceeds that of individual members and enables individuals to learn more rapidly. Svensson[29] offers a negotiated order framework where structural constraints and local negotiation processes continually feedback and evolve. Economic evaluation adopts an approach which is rational and explicit by comparing resource implications and benefits of alternative ways of delivering healthcare.

Although historically the development of doctor/nurse skill mix has occurred ahead of evidence of effectiveness, there is a developing literature to suggest that in some areas, substituting nurses for doctors gives equal or better health outcomes. However, there remains little evidence of cost effectiveness at a time when skill mix changes are being introduced in an effort to increase health service efficiency. Unfortunately, the debate remains characterised by rhetoric and historical precedent, and a recent edition of the *British Medical Journal* focusing on the area concluded it to be 'a bit of a muddle'.

Perspectives which include power, status and gender retain a considerable influence on skill mix changes, and health professionals may be reluctant to relinquish their traditional roles. Developments take place against a background of limited room for manoeuvre and extended lead times due to the long training requirements of health professionals. There is also the danger that analysing skill mix from a limited economic perspective will overlook differences that might not be revealed in an economic evaluation yet may be important in practice.

In summary, there are a number of problems in applying economic evaluation to the development of skill mix, and we have argued that in many cases the evidence base will not be accessible to enable an exact optimisation of skills. A pragmatic approach will be needed deriving solutions that are satisfactory rather than optimum, drawing on evidence where it is available but recognising its limitations and living with uncertainty when it is not. Nevertheless, there are a number of fundamental economic principles that can facilitate decisions and guard against the introduction of changes which are thought to be efficient when in fact they may not be so.

References

1   Department of Health (2000) *A Health Service of All the Talents: developing the NHS workforce. Consultation document on the review of workforce planning.* DoH, London.

2   Lewis R (2001) *Nurse Led Primary Care Learning from PMS Pilots.* King's Fund, London.

3   Stillwell B, Greenfield S, Drury M *et al.* (1987) A nurse practitioner in general practice: working style and pattern of consultation. *J R Coll Gen Pract.* **37:** 154–7.

4   Richardson G and Maynard A (1995) *Fewer Doctors? More Nurses? A Review of the Knowledge Base of Doctor/Nurse Substitution.* Discussion paper 135. University of York, York.

5   NHS Management Executive (1996) *Primary Care: delivering the future.* HMSO, London.

6   Rashid A, Watts A and Lenehan C (1996) Skill mix in primary care: sharing clinical workload and understanding professional roles. *Br J Gen Pract.* **6:** 639–40.

7   Freeling P (1981) Communication between doctors and nurses. In: J Walter and G McLachlan (eds) *Relationship and Prejudice.* Nuffield Provincial Hospital Trust, London.

8   Ratto M, Burgess S, Croxson B *et al.* (2001) *Team-Based Incentives in the NHS: an economic analysis.* CMPO Working Paper 01/37, Centre for Market and Public Organisation, University of Bristol, Bristol.

9   Wilson M, Ball JG, Banks IG *et al.* (1996) *Medical Workforce.* BMJ Books, London.

10   RCGP (1996) *The Nature of General Practice.* Report for General Practice 27. Royal College of General Practitioners, London.

11   DHSS (1986) *Neighbourhood Nursing: a focus for care.* DHSS, London.

12   Casey N and Smith R (1997) Bringing nurses and doctors closer together. *BMJ.* **314:** 617–18.

13   Department of Health (2000) *The NHS Plan.* DoH, London.

14   Drummond M (1994) *Economic Analysis Alongside Control Trials.* DoH, London.

15   Jenkins-Clarke S, Carr-Hill R, Dixon P and Pringle M (1997) *Skill Mix in Primary Care.* Centre for Health Economics, University of York, York.

16   Kernick D, Reinhold D, Sawkins J *et al.* (2000) A cost-consequence study of a dermatology nurse in primary care. *Br J Gen Pract.* **50:** 555–9.

17   Hassell K, Whittington Z, Lantride J *et al.* (2001) Managing demand: transfer of management of self limiting illness to community pharmacies. *BMJ.* **323:** 146–7.

18   Kernick DP (2000) Costs are as important as outcomes (Letter). *BMJ.* **321:** 567.

19   Graham B and McGregor K (1997) What does a GP consultation cost? *Br J Gen Pract.* **47:** 170–2.

20   Netten A, Dennett J and Knight J (1999) *Unit Cost of Health and Social Care.* PSSRU, University of Kent, Kent.

21   Ryan M and Shackley P (1995) Assessing the benefits of health care: how far should we go? *Qual Health Care.* **4:** 207–13.

22   Orchard C (1994) Comparing health outcomes. *BMJ.* **308:** 1493–6.

23   Wilson-Barnet J and Beech S (1994) Evaluating the clinical nurse specialist: a review. *Int J Nurse Studies.* **31(6):** 561–71.

24   Mauskopf J, Paul J, Grant J and Stergachis A (1998) The role of cost-consequence analysis in healthcare decision making. *Pharmacoeconomics.* **13(3):** 277–88.

25 Spitzer WO, Sackett DL, Sibley JC *et al.* (1974) The Burlington randomised trial of a nurse practitioner. *NEJM.* **290:** 251–6.

26 Torgerson DJ and Spencer A (1996) Marginal costs and benefits. *BMJ.* **312:** 35–6.

27 Pratt J, Gordon P and Plamping D (2000) *Working Whole Systems: putting theory into practice in organisations.* King's Fund, London.

28 Senge P (1990) *The Fifth Disciple: the art and practice of the learning organisation.* Double Day Publishers, New York.

29 Svennson R (1996) The interplay between doctors and nurses – a negotiated order perspective. *Sociology Health Illness.* **18:** 379–8.

CHAPTER 15

Economic evaluation of shifts in services from secondary to primary care

David Kernick and Anthony Scott

The continuing emphasis on a primary care led NHS is likely to encourage a shift of services from secondary to primary care. However, there are difficulties in obtaining evidence of cost effectiveness of these shifts, and there is a danger that the transfer of services may be assumed to be efficient when in fact they may not be so.

This chapter outlines some of the problems encountered when shifting services across the secondary/primary care interface from an economic perspective, and highlights some of the barriers to progress in this area.

Key points
- The continuing emphasis on a primary care led NHS is encouraging a shift of services from secondary to primary care.
- There is a limited evidence base of effectiveness and cost effectiveness complicated by methodological problems when undertaking research in this area.
- Due to high capital costs there may be difficulties disinvesting from secondary care.
- Cultural differences between the two systems can make shifts difficult. Decision makers should have realistic expectations of the difficulties involved.
- The incentive mechanisms that direct GP behaviour in this area are poorly understood.
- There is a danger that shifts may occur which are thought to be efficient when in fact they may not be so.

- Policy makers should have realistic expectations of the difficulties involved in changing services rather than being surprised and overwhelmed by them.
- Attention should be focused on improving efficiency at the interface through cooperation and communication, rather than shifting services across it.

Chapter sections
- **Introduction**
- **Problems with shifting services from secondary to primary care**
- **Conclusion**

Introduction

Economic analysis offers a framework to compare the costs and benefits of different interventions to assist decision makers in effective allocation of limited resources. From the broader NHS perspective, shifts between secondary and primary care aim to maximise the health of the population from a fixed healthcare budget.

Over the past decade there has been an increasing emphasis on expanding primary care. Although growth of this sector has occurred, large differences in

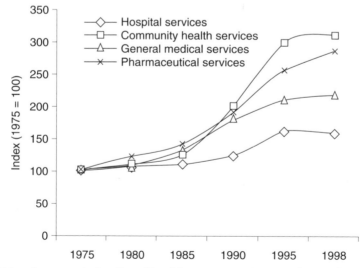

Figure 15.1:   Increases in funding of healthcare sectors (source: *Compendium of Health Statistics* (13e) (2001) Office of Health Economics, London).

funding between secondary and primary care remain (Figure 15.1). Previous work identified that the main source of growth in expenditure in primary care was an increasing share of new 'growth' money, with expenditure on secondary care remaining relatively stable.[1] This shift in the balance of expenditure between sectors does not necessarily lead to substitution.

Four types of shift can be recognised:

- physical relocation of services (e.g. physiotherapy, consultant outreach clinics)
- direct access by GPs to hospital facilities (e.g. ultrasound investigation)
- total care shifts (e.g. minor surgery, near patient testing, hospital at home schemes)
- partial care shifts (e.g. early hospital discharge, chronic disease shared care).

Incentives to shift the balance of care towards the primary sector were first introduced in the 1990 GP contract.[2] This identified core services which were to be directed by financial incentive, some of which had implications for a shift in services from secondary care. Minor surgery and the emphasis on health promotion and chronic disease management were particularly important in this respect. However, the cost effectiveness of these shifts were unproven. Scott and Maynard[3] called this reform 'a shot in the dark' and cautioned that without proper evaluation GPs may have been induced to practice inefficiently.

GP fundholding provided additional incentives to increase the range of practice-based services but measurable changes were small.[4] Despite a limited evidence base and methodological shortcomings in existing studies,[5] the government remained committed to an expansion of primary care based on the principles of efficiency and evidence-based practice.[6] Since GP fundholding was abolished in 1997, primary care continues to dominate resource allocation decisions in the form of primary care groups or trusts. These continuing developments have emphasised the role of patient representatives and healthcare professionals in higher level decision making, rather than explicit incentives to encourage shifts in the balance of care.

Box 15.1: Some factors influencing a shift of services towards primary care

- Financial incentive for GPs to provide additional services associated with GP purchasing.
- Long secondary care waiting lists.
- A perception that primary care services contain costs.
- Primary care practitioners may be better placed to assess need and improve services.
- May facilitate patient involvement in the delivery of healthcare.

Nevertheless, there continue to be major changes in the balance of care as services are modernised and redesigned influenced by factors shown in Box 15.1. However, unless the economic issues on secondary to primary shifts are thought through clearly, there is a danger that shifts may occur which are thought to be efficient when in fact they may not be so.

Problems with shifting services from secondary to primary care

Shifts in services are usually characterised by changes in the location in which care takes place, but can also involve changes in the professional delivering the services. They may arise as new resources become available, be financed by the withdrawal of secondary care resources or a combination of both. How an economic evaluation is undertaken will depend on the aim of the exercise and different results may be obtained for different situations. For example, if a hospital at home service is an additional service using additional resources with the aim of meeting increased demand, the aim will be to allocate these new resources efficiently. Alternatively, where hospital at home is intended to replace current care by releasing existing hospital resources, due to the high fixed cost of secondary care there will have to be a certain threshold size for the new service before resources can actually be released (i.e. release secondary care staff time or ward closure). Decision makers must be clear about their aims, the scope of the shift and the perspective of the economic exercise – who is asking the question and why?

Problems identifying suitable shifts

Difficulties in evaluating both the scale and appropriateness of shifts can result from ambiguity of definitions of secondary and primary care, and of the nature of shifts between them.[1] It has been argued that as an antecedent to any assessment, the heterogeneous list of primary care characteristics should be resolved into a short list of attributes which are well defined, robust, comprehensive and exclusive. Direct access, generalist care, longitudinal care and delivery in a community setting are the elements suggested.[5] Using this definition, transfers from hospitals to institutional settings such as community hospitals are not seen as shifts to the primary care sector.

This simplistic analysis may overlook a more fundamental cultural difference between the two sectors. Culture can be seen as a common way of making sense

Table 15.1:   Some differences between secondary and primary care

Perspective	Secondary care	Primary care
Financial organisation	Salaried medical contractors, no financial incentives, no personal risk	Independent medical contractors, financial incentives, personal financial risk
Service attributes	Single speciality	Continuous, comprehensive and coordinated care
Access	Indirect	Direct
Setting	Hospital based	Community based
Decision making	High levels of certainty, explicit, driven by scientific evidence	Low level of certainty, decisions often implicit, mediate between social, psychological and scientific evidence

of systems – the way things are understood, organised, judged and valued,[7] and it has been suggested that if shifts are to be secured, a cultural change will be required among both the profession and the public.[8] Understanding the broader cultural characteristics of each system rather than a limited set of attributes may offer greater insight into where efficient shifts in services may be located. Some of these characteristics are shown in Table 15.1.

Methodological problems in evaluating shifts

The methodological difficulties of evaluating effectiveness and cost effectiveness in this area are well recognised,[1,5,9] and stakeholders have expressed concern over the lack of a reliable evidence base.[10]

Lack of comprehensive cost data

Quality and comprehensiveness of cost data remain major issues. For example, increasing attention will need to be paid to the costs falling on patients, carers and social services. Problems are likely to arise from omission of important elements of costs relevant in one context but not another. For example, studies of early hospital discharge should include living costs at home over the study period, as hospital costs will include living expenses of an inpatient.

Failure to capture relevant opportunity cost

When measuring resources in economic terms, the objective is to identify the opportunity cost – what is being foregone in order to provide a service. First, an accurate identification of the opportunity cost of GP time should be carefully considered – what is the GP having to release to take up new activity? Second, the use of secondary care released capacity should be identified. For example, a release in hospital bed occupancy due to earlier discharge to primary care may result in high levels of activity and reduced waiting lists rather than true cost savings.

Undertaking a marginal analysis

In many cases the question is not whether or not to provide a service but how much to provide. As the relationship between resources invested and benefits incurred is rarely a straight line, the importance of undertaking a marginal analysis should always be recognised – how do benefits change with incremental shifts in resources? In most cases, benefits cannot be tested over a range of resource investments, and an attempt should be made to define the most relevant incremental analysis to perform based on the context of the exercise.

Capturing outcomes of service shifts

When undertaking an economic analysis, ideally outcomes should be described in a single measure to allow comparisons to be made. However, shifts in care will encompass a range of measures that will include clinical outcomes, health status, changes in quality of life and patient satisfaction. Non-health benefits such as improved access and waiting times are also important. Some of these measures may improve, while some may get worse. A further complication is the relative importance that patients place on these attributes. For example, would a patient trade-off a shorter waiting time for better access? These problems are considered in more detail in Chapter 21. Even with these broader outcomes, studies may fail to capture the implications of service shifts adequately. Other attributes of practice workload such as increased stress may be overlooked.

In most cases, a single measure of outcome will be insufficient to capture changes in service shifts, and a cost consequence approach may be the best approach. This presents a wide range of outcome variables to be assessed in a disaggregated form allowing decision makers to apply their own judgements on the relative merits of each benefit (*see* Chapter 11). Table 15.2 shows how a cost consequence study of the transference of gastroscopy services to primary care might appear.

Table 15.2:   A theoretical example of a cost consequence study – transferring gastroscopy services to primary care

Costs	Consequences
GP and nurse (what activity is being given up by these practitioners to undertake the new service?)	Health state
	Diagnostic accuracy
Saving in hospital resources (what is being released and how is it being utilised?)	Patient satisfaction (better access, shorter waiting times, understanding of condition)
Capital costs (e.g new buildings, equipment)	Patient dissatisfaction (lack of expert care)
Patient costs	Patient pathway through system until final clinical outcome
Costs of administering primary care service including quality control	Loss of opportunities for secondary care training

Problems with generalisability

Economic evaluation cannot always be generalised in ways similar to the results of clinical trials.[11] In such a complex area as the secondary/primary care interface, economic evaluation will be highly context dependent. Different geographical areas will have their unique local histories, interests, contingencies and cost data. For example, a review of studies comparing hospital care at home with standard hospital care found quite different results due to different contextual elements.[9] A review of new patient testing in primary care found that many new diagnostic technologies were disappointing in practice due to a failure to address setting specific issues that were not apparent during their evaluation.[12] There will also be dangers of extrapolating results obtained from short trial periods to longer time horizons, particularly in a service area that is changing rapidly.

Difficulties in releasing resources in secondary care

Efficiency is not the only criterion which directs health service activity. Other institutional considerations may be relevant which can include responding to organisational reward structures, the maximisation of personal well being and pursuit of the quiet life.[13] In a review of the practical use of economic techniques to inform resource allocation decisions across the secondary/primary care interface, McIver *et al.*[14] noted the strength of established interests. Opportunities to make changes were mainly at the margins. Major disinvestment barriers arose from the relatively high proportion of fixed costs in secondary care and the difficulties in identifying how much money had been saved following the introduction of service change. Disinvestment creates losers whether in terms of loss of income, loss of role or agency survival.

Barriers in primary care

The factors that influence GPs' behaviour in terms of both financial and non-financial incentives are poorly understood.[15] Against a background of increasing pressure on GPs from many areas, their ability to accommodate new services from secondary care may be limited, and currently there is little support for new roles for GPs that accompany shifts to primary care.[16] Even with the development of an evidence base GPs do not necessarily follow evidence-based guidelines,[17] and there may be a dissonance between findings derived from research settings and the experience of GPs themselves.

Finally, lack of leadership in primary care has been highlighted as a major concern in developing service shifts.[10] Initiatives often involve a number of agencies in an area characterised by structural tension in the distribution of power and authority. This may change with the development of multiagency primary care trusts, which challenge old working practices with their broader managerial and financial perspectives.

Conclusion

Current policy making remains firmly in line with the development of a primary care led NHS underpinned by evidence of effectiveness and cost effectiveness. However, the evidence base to support shifts remains limited and there are many methodological difficulties. Research resources are also limited and have an opportunity cost. For example, over the last eight years, the NHS Research and Development Executive has commissioned 70 projects at a cost of £8 million (www.doh.gov.uk/ntrd/rd/psi/intro.htm), but these focus on a limited number of areas. Studies cannot be undertaken in all clinical areas that will be generalisable in both location and time across a rapidly changing NHS. There are also more fundamental methodological concerns. The organisation of healthcare is complex and changes in one part of the system, however small, can induce disproportional and unintended changes in other parts of the system, which can easily be overlooked. Analysing such complex systems by reduction into their component parts may not always provide the right answers (*see* Chapter 30).

Undoubtedly, successful shifts between secondary and primary care have already occurred. For example, physiotherapy clinics, where disinvestment was not a major issue, have been shifted with little or no resistance. Many practices are running anticoagulation clinics and specialist outreach sessions. However, in most cases it has not been possible to identify the resource implications of existing shifts which may have actually encouraged inefficient use of resources. For example, the development of minor surgery in primary care may have encouraged treatment of patients who would not have otherwise been treated and made only a minor impact on hospital workload.[18]

It is important to recognise that shifts in the balance of care are part of an overall process of integration that occurs at a number of levels.[19] For example, a service will be more integrated if it is jointly managed or financed, or if communication is enhanced, even though no change in the location of care or the professional delivering it has occurred. This seems to be more relevant in an era of enhancing cooperation and removing organisational boundaries in the NHS. Couching organisational change in terms of shifting services between primary and secondary care only serves to highlight the differences between them, thus reinforcing their boundaries.

Box 15.2:   Some questions to ask when undertaking secondary/primary care shifts

- What is the aim of the service being delivered?
- Is a shift in service an option in improving service delivery?
- If so, is the shift acceptable to all stakeholders?
- Is there an evidence base for the proposed shift which captures all the relevant costs and outcomes?
- What are the local cost implications?
- What are the local values placed on the potential changes in outcome (clinical and non-clinical)?
- What seems the best increment in service shift to undertake?
- Are new resources available or is disinvestment required from secondary care?
- If disinvestment is to be undertaken from secondary care and this is a practical option can the released resources be identified?
- Are there implications for other services that may have been overlooked?
- How practical is it to implement the proposed change and what is the cost of initiating the change?

Innovations in service shifts may have a better chance of success when additional resources are available, but the danger remains that services may be introduced that are thought to be efficient when in fact they may not be so. Perhaps the best way forward is to acknowledge that optimal solutions are rarely obtainable. It is important to have realistic expectations of the difficulties involved in changing services, rather than being surprised and overwhelmed by them and to recognise that there may be only limited scope for manoeuvre. Box 15.2 shows some relevant questions to ask when undertaking shifts. However, we conclude by suggesting that the initial effort should focus on efficient management of the interface (e.g. improving communication, joint protocols) between the two systems rather than shifting services between them.

References

1 Miller P, Craig N, Scott A, Walker A and Hanlon P (1999) Measuring progress towards a primary care led NHS. *Br J Gen Pract*. **49**: 451–5.
2 Department of Health (1989) *General Practice and the National Health Service: the 1990 contract*. HMSO, London.
3 Scott T and Maynard A (1991) *Will the New GP Contract Lead to Cost Effective Medical Practice?* Discussion paper 82. Centre for Health Economics, University of York, York.
4 Mays N, Mulligan J and Goodwin N (2000) The British quasi-market in healthcare: a balance sheet of the evidence. *J Health Service Res Policy*. **5(1)**: 49–58.
5 Godbere E, Robinson R and Steiner A (1997) Economic evaluation and the shifting balance towards primary care: definitions, evidence and methodological issues. *Health Economics*. **6**: 275–94.
6 NHSE (1996) *Primary Care: the future*. NHS Executive, Leeds.
7 Davies H and Mannion R (2000) Organisational culture and quality of healthcare. *Qual Healthcare*. **9**: 111–19.
8 Coulter A (1995) Shifting the balance from secondary to primary care. *BMJ*. **311**: 1447–8.
9 Coast J, Hensher M, Mulligan J, Shepperd S and Jones J (2000) Conceptual and practical difficulties with the economic evaluation of Health Service developments. *J Health Service Res Policy*. **5**: 142–8.
10 O'Cathain A, Musson G and Munro J (1999) Shifting services from secondary to primary care: stakeholders' views of the barriers. *J Health Service Res Policy*. **4**: 154–60.
11 Bryan S and Brown J (1998) Extrapolation of cost effectiveness information to local settings. *J Health Services Res Policy*. **3**: 108–13.
12 Delaney B, Wilson S, Fitzmaurice D, Hyde C and Hobbs R (2000) New patient tests in primary care: setting the standards for evaluation. *J Health Res Policy*. **5**: 37–41.
13 Jan S (2000) Institutional considerations in priority setting: transactions cost perspective on PBMA. *Health Economics*. **9**: 631–41.
14 McIver S, Baines D, Ham C and McCleod H (2000) *Setting Priorities and Managing Demands in the NHS*. Health Services Management Centre, University of Birmingham, Birmingham.

15 Scott A (1996) Primary or secondary care: what can economics contribute to evaluation at the interface? *J Public Health Med.* **18:** 19–26.

16 Miller P, Scott A and Vale L (1998) Increased general practice workload due to a primary care led NHS: the need for evidence to support rhetoric. *Br J Gen Practice.* **48:** 1085–8.

17 Salisbury C, Bosanquet N, Williamson E *et al.* (1998) The implementation of evidence based medicine in general practice prescribing. *Br J Gen Pract.* **48:** 1849–51.

18 Lowy A, Brazier J, Fall M, Thomas K, Jones N and Williams B (1993) Minor surgery by general practitioners under the 1990 Contract: effects on the hospital workload. *BMJ.* **307:** 413–7.

19 Simoens S (2002) *The Dimensions and Determinants of Integration in Primary Care.* PhD Thesis, University of Aberdeen, Aberdeen.

CHAPTER 16

Applying economic evaluation to complementary and alternative medicine

David Kernick and Adrian White

Despite the popularity of complementary and alternative medicine with the public, it enjoys little provision within the NHS. With the demise of fundholding and increasing pressure on budgets, there is unlikely to be any expansion in this area unless evidence of cost effectiveness can be obtained. This chapter reviews current evidence in this area and outlines the difficulties of obtaining economic data to inform commissioners.

Key points
- Complementary and alternative therapies reflect a diverse range of interventions.
- The emphasis is on illness – what the patient experiences, rather than disease – and what the health professional recognises.
- Evidence of effectiveness is scarce and there is no valid evidence of cost effectiveness.
- There are a number of difficulties undertaking research in this area to inform purchasing decisions.
- Complementary and alternative medicine cannot be excluded from rigorous evaluation, but may open a broader agenda about the meaning of health.

Chapter sections
- Introduction
- What is complementary and alternative medicine?
- The use of complementary and alternative medicine in the UK
- Current evidence of cost effectiveness of CAM
- Undertaking CAM research to inform purchasing decisions
- Conclusion

Introduction

The popularity of complementary and alternative medicine (CAM) has increased dramatically over the past 20 years and in the US, more patients visit complementary therapists than orthodox doctors.[1] In the UK, over 13% of adults visit CAM therapists in any one year,[2] but CAM retains only a small presence within the NHS. With increasing pressure on budgets, CAM is unlikely to displace orthodox medicine unless evidence of cost effectiveness can be obtained. This chapter reviews the current evidence of cost effectiveness and the difficulties of undertaking economic evaluation in this area.

What is complementary and alternative medicine?

One of the problems of CAM evaluation is that its therapies reflect a diverse range of interventions that often overlap. A House of Lords' report[3] pragmatically divided CAM into three categories as shown in Box 16.1.

Box 16.1:   Categories of CAM disciplines

Group 1: Professionally organised alternative therapies
Acupuncture, chiropractic, herbal medicine, homoeopathy and osteopathy.

Group 2: Complementary therapies
Alexander technique, aromatherapy, Bach and other flower remedies, bodywork therapies including massage, counselling stress therapy, hypnotherapy, meditation, reflexology, shiatsu, healing, Maharishi Ayurvedic medicine, nutritional medicine and yoga.

Group 3: Alternative disciplines
- Long-established and traditional systems of healthcare
  Anthroposophical medicine, Ayurvedic medicine, Chinese herbal medicine, Eastern medicine (Tibb), naturopathy and traditional Chinese medicine.
- Other alternative disciplines
  Crystal therapy, dowsing, iridology, kinesiology and radionics.

In general, CAM reflects a more holistic approach to care than orthodox medicine and emphasises illness (what the patient experiences) rather than disease (what the traditional healthcare system recognises).[4] Some distinguishing features are:

- mental, physical and spiritual aspects of the person are emphasised and seen as interdependent
- symptoms are assessed in relation to an individual patient rather than by applying a disease framework
- emphasis is on chronic disorders
- a recognition of the importance of self-empowerment and self-healing.

Therapeutic modalities include the quality of the therapeutic interaction, philosophical congruence between practitioner and patient, and an acceptable illness model which helps patients understand their predicament.[5] The suggestion is that CAM influences the broader elements of psychological, social and physical factors that influence the illness experience.

The use of complementary and alternative medicine in the UK

A large stratified population survey estimated that 13.6% of UK adults had visited a CAM therapist in a 12-month period.[2] Five homoeopathic hospitals exist with the NHS and a survey of 964 GP practices found that 40% provided

Table 16.1: Population estimates of use and expenditure on complementary and alternative medicine in a 12-month period, UK 1998[2]

	Estimated total visits per year (million)	Estimated personal expenditure (£ million)	Estimated NHS visits (million)	Estimated NHS expenditure (£ million)
Acupuncture	3.1	47	1.02	25.9
Chiropractic	7.5	160	0.36	8.2
Homoeopathy	1.3	31	0.12	3.3
Hypnotherapy	1.2	34	0.14	5.3
Medical herbalism	1.5	31	–	–
Osteopathy	7.3	147	0.45	10.1
Reflexology	4.3	47	0.19	3.1
Aromatherapy	6.2	84	–	–
Total	31.7	581	2.31	55.9

some form of access to CAM.[6] In half of these practices, a member of the primary care team provided the services, and the most frequent therapies offered were homoeopathy and acupuncture. It has been estimated that 10% of physiotherapists use acupuncture in their work and acupuncture is often a feature of local pain clinic services. However, the availability of CAM is haphazard and poorly integrated into orthodox medicine. Its provision is dependent on the enthusiasm of NHS staff and is vulnerable to the politics of local funding. It has diminished since the demise of fundholding. Estimates of use and expenditure on CAM are shown in Table 16.1.

Current evidence of cost effectiveness of CAM

Systematic reviews have highlighted the lack of rigour in the majority of clinical effectiveness studies. These include lack of statistical power, poor controls, inconsistency of treatment, difficulty in identifying appropriate placebo interventions and lack of standardisation of interventions.[7] Research design is often confounded by the lack of standardisation and overlap of many types of CAM.

A systematic review of economic evaluations of CAM identified a total of 34 studies, which fell into two general groups[8] – those that investigated the effects of providing a range of CAM and those that analysed a single therapy. Manipulative therapy for back pain received the most attention, presumably due to the economic impact of this problem (Table 16.2). One large randomised study for back pain comparing chiropractic clinics with hospital outpatient management concluded that savings of £9.4 million per annum were gained in industrial output and reduction in sickness benefit payments.[9] One retrospective study[10] suggested that targeted acupuncture might reduce referral costs for musculoskeletal problems. There were serious methodological deficiencies in every study. All trials were undertaken from a limited economic perspective and were not performed according to established guidelines for economic evaluation. It was concluded that findings were contradictory and of little value to purchasers.

Undertaking CAM research to inform purchasing decisions

The NHS is committed to providing 'a comprehensive range of services that are clinically appropriate and cost effective',[15] but the research process itself has an

Table 16.2:   Controlled trials of manipulative therapies for back pain with basic economic evaluation

Reference	Setting and subjects (n)	Comparative interventions	Outcomes
Meade et al.[9]	Back pain (721)	• Chiropractic clinic • Hospital outpatients	Chiropractic greater symptom relief at follow-up, and more cost effective
Timm[11]	Chronic back pain (250)	• Physical therapy • Joint manipulation • Home exercise • Apparatus exercise • Standard care	Exercise regimens significantly greater benefit and more cost effective
Carey et al.[12]	Self-referred back pain – patients, not randomised (1555)	• Chiropractic • Orthopaedic surgeon • Primary care physician • Health maintenance organisation	No difference in recovery of function – orthopaedic and chiropractic most expensive; less medication, greater satisfaction with chiropractic
Cherkin et al.[13]	Acute low back pain in primary care (321)	• Chiropractic • Physiotherapy • Education booklet	More residual dysfunction in booklet group; medical costs considerably lower in booklet group
Skargren et al.[14]	Acute low back pain in primary care (323)	• Chiropractic • Physiotherapy	No difference in costs or benefits

opportunity cost. Four criteria for prioritising research opportunities have been identified:[7]

• extent of use of an intervention by the public
• the importance of the condition being treated
• feasibility of conducting the research
• quantity and quality of available preliminary data to help determine the most appropriate type of research.

The popularity of CAM may indicate that the public is sending a message about the kind of treatment they want but are not receiving. This message may receive support from the fact that, despite increases in health spending, stratified annual household surveys show that the number of people describing themselves in poor health continues to increase.[16] Patients seem to be concerned about how services are provided in addition to the end result. It is often the issues of humanity, dignity, therapeutic relationships, communication, mutual respect, trust and availability that concern them.[17] These are issues that are relatively under-researched and hard to quantify for economic analysis.

CAM opens a broader agenda about the meaning of health and what is important to the patient. People often look for hope, reassurance, encouragement, understanding, explanation and information, as well as treatment. Patients may value an evaluation framework which encompasses an ethic of care emphasising relationships, validation of illness and the importance of therapeutic interaction – outcomes overlooked in formal economic studies. Meenan[18] has suggested that the benefits of CAM will not necessarily be reflected in the restrictive conceptual framework of the QALY. The methodology is simply too insensitive to the values of patients or the broader community to inform policy meaningfully in this area. He concludes that explorations of the cost effectiveness of CAM present health economists with remarkable opportunities to explore the meaning of health, utility and well being to the patient and the community.

The significance of process and the argument for a reconceptualisation of health to inform clinical and economic research and policy clearly extend beyond CAM and into conventional care. Health economists are beginning to accept this challenge with the recognition of the importance of the benefit gained from the process of care[19] and the accommodation of other insights obtained from qualitative research.[20]

Conclusion

Unfortunately, the CAM field remains heavily dependent on anecdote and clinical impression, and there is even an absence of basic studies that could identify the most promising areas to research. A major problem is the poor research culture of CAM with virtually no infrastructure and only one dedicated university department in the UK. However, research methodology is being introduced in CAM training, and in the US a National Center for Complementary and Alternative Medicine has been established to explore the area using rigorous scientific methodology.

Nevertheless, despite the lack of evidence of clinical effectiveness CAM often does achieve higher satisfaction levels than orthodox medicine. Much of this satisfaction is likely to be due to process attributes that are unlikely to be detected using existing measures. It could be argued that it is illness and not disease that dictates economic activity and social functioning. For example, in chronic back pain it is recognised that function has no relationship to clinical findings.[21]

Patients are clearly giving the message about the kind of treatment they want. CAM cannot be excluded from rigorous evaluation and unless cost effectiveness estimates are developed, its provision will ultimately be eroded with increasing pressure on existing resources. When viewed through the current decision-making framework, there is as yet no case for the integration of CAM into the NHS. However, the subject may open a broader agenda about health and what is meaningful to the patient, offering new challenges to health economists to develop frameworks that reflect more closely the pragmatic requirements of the population and healthcare practitioners.

References

1 Eisenberg DM, Davis R *et al.* (1998) Trends in alternative medicine use in the United States 1990–1997. *JAMA.* **280:** 1569–75.

2 Thomas KJ, Nicholl JP and Coleman P (2001) Use and expenditure on complementary medicine in England: a population based survey. *Complement Ther Med.* **9:** 2–11.

3 House of Lords Select Committee on Science and Technology (2000) *Complementary and Alternative Medicine.* HMSO, London.

4 Evans RG and Stoddart GL (1990) Producing health, consuming healthcare. *Social Science Med.* **31:** 1347–63.

5 Stevinson C (2001) Why patients use complementary and alternative medicine. In: E Ernst, M Pittler, C Stevinson and A White (eds) *The Desktop Guide to Complementary and Alternative Medicine.* Mosby, London, 395–403.

6 Thomas KJ, Nicholl JP and Fall M (2001) Access to complementary medicine via general practice. *Br J Gen Pract.* **51:** 25–30.

7 Nahin R and Straus S (2001) Research into complementary and alternative medicine: problems and potential. *BMJ.* **322:** 161–4.

8 White AR and Ernst E (2000) Economic analysis of complementary medicine: a systematic review. *Complement Ther Med.* **8:** 111–18.

9 Meade TW, Dyer S, Browne W *et al.* (1995) Randomised comparison of chiropractic and hospital outpatients management for low back pain: results from extended follow up. *BMJ.* **311:** 349–51.

10 Lindall S (1999) Is acupuncture for pain relief in general practice cost-effective? *Acupunct Med.* **17:** 97–100.

11 Timm KE (1994) A randomised controlled study of active and passive treatments for chronic low back pain. *J Orthop Sports Phys Ther.* **20:** 276–86.

12 Carey TS, Garrett J, Jackman A *et al.* (1995) The outcomes and costs of care for acute low back pain among patients seen by primary care practitioners, chiropractors, and orthopaedic surgeons. The North Carolina Back Pain Project. *NEJM.* **333:** 913–17.

13 Cherkin DC, Deyo RA, Battie M *et al.* (1998) A comparison of physical therapy, chiropractic manipulation, and provision of an educational booklet for the treatment of patients with low back pain. *NEJM.* **339:** 1021–9.

14 Skargren EI, Carlsson PG and Oberg BE (1998) One-year follow-up comparison of the cost and effectiveness of chiropractic and physiotherapy as primary management for back pain. *Spine.* **23:** 1875–84.

15 Department of Health (2000) *The NHS Plan: a plan for investment, a plan for reform.* HMSO, London.

16 *General Household Survey 1998* (1999) HMSO, London.

17 Mitchell A and Cormack M (1998) *Therapeutic Relationship in Complementary Healthcare.* Churchill Livingstone, London.

18 Meenan R (2001) Developing appropriate measures of the benefits of complementary and alternative medicine. *J Health Service Res Policy.* **6(1):** 38–43.

19 Ryan M and Shackley P (1995) Assessing the benefits of healthcare: how far should we go? *Qual Health Care.* **4:** 207–13.

20 Coast J (1999) The appropriate use of qualitative methods in health economics. *Health Economics.* **8:** 345–53.

21 Waddell G (1992) Biopsychosocial analysis of low back pain. *Clin Rheumatol.* **6:** 523–7.

CHAPTER 17

Using economic evaluation at grass roots level

Ruth McDonald and David Kernick

The large volume of economic evaluations published annually contrasts with the paucity of evidence relating to their impact on policy making. This chapter considers why this might be and argues that there are real barriers to the application of economic evaluation to decision making that cannot be resolved by increased data collection or methodological refinements. It suggests that health economists should work more closely with decision makers at all levels of the health service in order to understand more clearly the context of the environment in which decisions are made.

Key points
- The large volume of economic evaluations published annually contrasts with the paucity of evidence relating to their impact on policy making.
- Economic evaluation is underpinned by the rational model of decision-making which assumes proactive decision making and requires clarity of objectives and the ability to evaluate all options in detail.
- The rational approach contrasts with the day-to-day reactive environment of NHS decision making, where objectives may conflict and cause and effect relationships are often poorly understood.
- Implicit rationing and goal conflict result in inequalities in service delivery. This undermines the equity goals of the health system, but paradoxically maintains the system within limited resources.
- Pragmatic approaches to economic evaluation are being developed but health economists need to work more closely with those they seek to influence.

Chapter sections
- Introduction
- Health economic theory and health service reality: understanding the decision making context
- Problems with using economic information in practice
- Conclusion

Introduction

The volume of published economic evaluations is growing rapidly and over the next decade, health economics will exert an increasing influence on decision makers at all levels in healthcare. The UK NHS Economic Evaluation Database was established in 1995 by the NHS Research and Development programme to identify papers reporting economic evaluations, and contains over 5000 records. However, little is known about the influence of such studies on decision making at grassroots level. The limited evidence that is available suggests that to date, impact has been minimal. For example, in a review of the literature in 1993, Coyle[1] found that the impact of economic evaluations in the form of directly influencing healthcare decision making was difficult to detect. In this chapter we review why this might be.

Health economic theory and health service reality: understanding the decision making context

Decision making in healthcare is not always straightforward. Here we identify two contrasting frameworks.

Rational decision making

Economic evaluation is characterised by the rational model of decision making which involves the following steps:

- define and rank your values
- specify your objective (which will be compatible with these values)
- identify all relevant options for achieving the objective
- calculate the costs and consequences for each of these
- choose the option which will maximise the values you defined as important at the start of the process.

This approach characterises the 'sunny uplands' within healthcare and its top-down analysis. The focus is on optimisation and explicit recognition of values. This raises the question of whose values are to count in the process and how explicitly these can be stated, given the need to avoid bad publicity and the requirements of the political election cycle.

Economists commenting on barriers to the use of health economics at local level have tended to highlight the lack of information available to decision makers.[2] The suggestion is that more and better evaluations must be conducted to fill this information gap and other barriers that relate to the decision making context are ignored. However, the barriers may go far beyond this.

Decision making by muddling through

Healthcare practitioners and managers live in the 'the swampy lowlands' (Table 17.1). Here, the world is not full of cosy certainties like evidence-based medicine and guidelines, but an environment of complexity, uncertainty and contingency with limited room for manoeuvre. Unlike the picture painted in the rational model, which focuses on a single objective, healthcare issues are mainly multi-dimensional. For practitioners, progress is made through pragmatic, adaptive methods, accommodating and implementing small changes that they consider as evolving and improving on current treatment.[3] Methods that aim at optimisation belie the problems of working in complex organisations where solutions are at best satisfactory.

'Street level bureaucrats' who occupy this world enjoy wide discretion in relation to many areas of their work, but are faced with a gap between the resources required to deliver optimal care and the reality of available budgets. To resolve these conflicts decision makers develop pragmatic coping strategies, which allow them to process patients through the system. For example, GPs may ignore guidelines or implement them selectively according to what works for them. Although these coping strategies may undermine the goals of the health system in terms of providing equal access to care, paradoxically, they maintain the system and allow the delivery of care within a fixed budget.[4]

Table 17.1:   Life in a parallel track health service

Sunny uplands	Swampy lowlands
Healthcare – a technical act	Healthcare – a personal and social act
An elevation of the quantifiable – decisions always explicit	Intuition is important – solutions are often implicit
The aim is to reduce uncertainty by the application of science	The aim is to tolerate uncertainty and to mediate between the directives of science and the predicament of the individual
Emphasis on performance appraisal	Emphasis on reflection
Emphasis on outcomes	A recognition that outcome measurement is inherently problematic
Knowledge is universal and pivotal	Knowledge is temporary, dynamic and problematic
Systems can be understood by breaking them down into their component parts	There is more to systems than a sum of the individual parts

Problems with using economic information in practice

There have been a limited number of studies on the impact of economic evaluation at health authority and primary care group level. Appendix 1 reviews the evidence to date, and highlights the problems of applying simple economic analyses in the complex world of NHS decision making. Before these are explored in more depth we describe a recent case study which explores the impact of economic evaluation in relation to cholesterol lowering drugs (statins) on a number of local decision makers at health authority (HA) and primary care group (PCG) level.[5]

Several economic evaluations based on evidence from large randomised trials illustrated that statins are cost effective in the treatment of patients with coronary heart disease. A government advisory body (the Standing Medical Advisory Committee) produced guidance which drew the attention of NHS decision makers to this cost effective technology and stated the categories of patients who would benefit most from these drugs. However, the Department of Health also made clear that there would be no new money for these drugs. How did decision makers use this economic evidence in practice?

- Case 1: One local HA produced a statins guideline despite the fact that it had no new money for this. It defended its actions precisely on the basis that regardless of the guideline, most GPs would continue to 'do their own thing' anyway. This begs the question 'so what is the objective of the guideline process?' The answer appears to be that there is no objective or that doing something feels better than doing nothing, even though the outcome may be the same in either case. Thus when faced with a new technology, this HA response has been to produce guidelines, but the purpose of the guidelines is not discussed.

- Case 2: A local PCG produced guidelines with little difficulty precisely because it did not specify objectives. Here, the aim was only to produce a statins guideline and the fact that no thought is given to monitoring its implementation supports this.
- Case 3: Attempts of another HA at more systematic decision making on statins using health economic analysis and locally relevant data required decision makers to specify their objectives. Staff were torn between wanting to encourage the uptake of this relatively cost effective drug and wanting to tightly restrict its use in order to balance budgets. Having acknowledged these tensions explicitly, decision makers were unable to construct a guideline, with the result that decision paralysis and inaction ensued. In this case, decision makers wanted to contain costs but at the same time, to encourage the uptake of statins, reduce inequalities in access to care but restrict the use of drugs to an 'affordable' level. They were unable to say what 'affordable' meant, as they had no new money and no potential for disinvesting from existing services. In private, some decision makers suggested that older patients should receive low priority for treatment. They argued that the public, when asked, always give priority to younger patients. However, these decision makers were not permitted to express such views in public. Explicitly stating values at the start of the process in the manner assumed by the rational model is often not possible in NHS contexts.

These studies showed that forcing decision makers to consider goal conflicts explicitly creates anguish on their part by exposing the gap between the rational ideal and reality. The HA which tried to use the economic evidence did not produce a statin guideline because the health economics input into the process laid bare the gap between 'rational' policy processes, in which objectives are clear and mutually consistent, and the real world context, in which objectives were ambiguous. Thus action is facilitated, and decision makers are happiest, if goals are not considered. However, this state of affairs is not a result of economic evaluation. Attempts to use economic evaluation merely serve to highlight the difficulty of rational approaches to resource allocation in a system where goals conflict and where many choices are informed by the exercise of implicit value judgements.

Health economists would argue that in order to pay for statins resources should be taken away from other, less cost effective, treatment areas. However,

HAs have at best, weak legitimacy for disinvesting from services, and the practical difficulties of removing or reducing existing services are well recognised. From these studies and the literature review we identify five difficulties that are encountered when economic information is used in practice.

Acquisition of evidence

In order to conduct an economic evaluation, evidence of effectiveness is required, but often obtaining this evidence is problematic. There are a number of practical problems that are well recognised, and although there is agreement on a number of basic principles governing the design of economic studies, many issues remain unresolved.[6] Disagreement can arise over method, presentation and interpretation,[7] or evidence can be interpreted selectively according to the interests of the evaluator. For example, two economic evaluations that were considered by NICE for the drug Orlistat[8] estimated a cost per QALY gained as £46,000 (range £19,000–£55,000) and £10,400 (range £8,400–£16,000). There was no overlap in the range of estimates from the two studies!

Pharmacoeconomic evaluations form the majority of published economic evaluations but many are commercially funded and like clinical trials can suffer from similar publication bias.[9] Table 17.2 shows the results of a study that compared the outcomes of pharmaceutical and non-pharmaceutical sponsors.

Poor presentation

Often studies are presented in ways that do not facilitate dissemination.[11] Results may be inaccessible to end users whose understanding of health economic principles is usually poor.

Table 17.2:   Publication bias in pharmaceutical studies[10]

	Pharmaceutical sponsor	Non-pharmaceutical sponsor
Conclusion favourable	60%	42%
Conclusion unfavourable	5%	36%
Overstatement of results	30%	13%

Problems with ambiguity

Ambiguity arises because goals conflict. Ambiguity is distinct from uncertainty where limitations to knowledge can be reduced by seeking information over time. When a situation is described as ambiguous a decision maker is less confident that any one thing is true, or that the world can be partitioned into mutually exclusive states. Health service decision makers face many objectives, such as increasing health gain, balancing budgets, minimising complaints and improving equality. No amount of additional information will resolve the lack of clarity between these conflicting elements.

Problems of power and legitimacy

In the NHS, healthcare decision making is no longer based on hierarchical relationships but networks, with the result that the policy process is one of governance as opposed to government. This means getting things done through other organisations. In order to implement policy decisions based on health economic evaluations, it is necessary to negotiate with and secure the cooperation of local stakeholders. As the objectives and values of these stakeholders may well conflict, this negotiation will not be easy. Decision makers may have limited powers over local stakeholders and cannot always apply top-down policy implementation. For example, clinicians can claim legitimacy when it comes to opposing any attempts to reduce services invoking their obligation of care to their patients.

Inflexible NHS finance regimen

The inflexibility of the NHS financial regimen is seen as a barrier to the implementation of health economic 'solutions' at local level. Finances are fixed and allocated annually. There is no provision for carrying forward resources from one year to the next, and health authorities are required to balance their budgets every year so that borrowing against future resources is not permitted. Until recently, transfers between budgets were not permissible but this has now been relaxed. For example, increased expenditure on drugs can be compensated from savings in the hospital budget, which gives decision makers a greater degree of flexibility. The impact of this change on decision makers is not yet clear.

Conclusion

Evidence to date has suggested that the impact of economic evaluation has not been commensurate with the volume of its literature. Where should health economists go from here? The first problem arises from a lack of understanding of the subject among commissioners, providers and patients who are becoming increasingly involved in decisions within the NHS. An educational campaign would be a useful first step.

Second, attempts by health economists to focus with increasing depth on small components of the healthcare system in isolation ignore the fact that when faced with complex systems, predictive and analytical power is often gained by standing back. Change in one aspect of a health system is likely to produce ripple effects throughout the rest of the system. Obtaining an understanding of these whole-system effects would seem preferable to increasing data acquisition and analysis on isolated aspects of the system.

Third, decision frameworks should be both accessible and acceptable to end users and reflect the context in which decisions are made. Technical fixes and mathematical models do not offer an easy escape from the conflicting values found in the healthcare environment.

Finally, and most importantly, health economists and those who commission and provide care should work more closely together. This implies that end users should participate in the construction of decision frameworks. The focus should be on pragmatic approaches that align the four key elements of health service research, economic evaluation, commissioning of care and service delivery around the day-to-day health and social problems of patients and practitioners.[12] This will require decision makers to be explicit about the values which inform their practice. Additionally, implicit in this approach is the recognition that trade-offs will be required between competing values held by different groups of stakeholders (e.g. GPs, PCT board, HAs, patients etc). If decision makers are to use economic evaluation to best effect, they need to find ways of involving local stakeholders in the process. In return, stakeholders must identify their values and make them transparent.

There are signs that the realities of the healthcare environment are being recognised by health economists and that the gap between rhetoric and reality is being bridged. For example, the importance of developing toolkits to facilitate economic evaluation rather than blindly following standardised methodology has been recognised.[13] Cost consequence analysis[14] emphasises the importance of presenting data on costs and benefits in dissaggregated form implying a recognition of the importance of value judgements from decision makers and an acceptance that benefits and disbenefits cannot always be condensed into a unitary output measure. The appropriate use of qualitative techniques in health economics has been described.[15] Finally, programme budgeting and marginal analysis[16] offers a pragmatic framework that can facilitate resource allocation by combining basic economic principles, available evidence and needs assessment. This approach is considered in more detail in the next chapter.

The gap between sunny uplands and swampy lowlands is diminishing, but there still remains some way to go.

References

1 Coyle D (1993) *Increasing the Impact of Economic Evaluation on Health Care Decision Making* (discussion paper 108). Centre for Health Economics, University of York, York.

2 Williams A (2000) Setting priorities: what is holding us back – inadequate information or inadequate institutions? In: A Coulter and C Ham (eds) *The Global Challenge of Health Care Rationing*. Open University Press, Buckingham.

3 Salisbury C, Bosanquet N, Wilkinson E *et al.* (1998) The implementation of evidence based medicine in general practice prescribing. *Br J Gen Prac.* **48:** 1849–51.

4 Lipsky M (1980) *Street-Level Bureaucracy*. Russell Sage, New York.

5 McDonald R (2000) *Using Health Economics in the NHS: case studies in local decision-making*. PhD Thesis. University of Liverpool, Liverpool.

6 Hutton J (1994) Economic evaluation of healthcare: a half way technology. *Health Economics.* **3:** 1–4.

7 Freemantle N and Maynard A (1994) Something rotten in the state of clinical and economic analysis. *Health Economics.* **3:** 63–7.

8 NICE (2000) *Guidance on the Use of Orlistat for the Treatment of Obesity in Adults*. NICE, London.

9 Sacristan J, Bolanos E, Hernadez J *et al.* (1997) Publication bias in health economic studies. *Pharmacoeconomics.* **11(3):** 289–90.

10 Friedman M, Saffron B and Stinson T (1999) Evaluation of conflict of interest in economic analyses of new drugs used in oncology. *JAMA.* **282(15):** 1453–7.

11 Mason J and Drummond M (1995) The Department of Health register of cost effectiveness studies: content and quality. *Health Trends.* **27:** 50–6.

12 Kernick DP, Stead J and Dixon M (1999) Time to refocus the academic effort (Editorial). *BMJ.* **319:** 206–7.

13 Drummond M, Brandt A, Luce B *et al.* (1993) Standardising methodologies for economic evaluation in healthcare: practice problems and potential. *Int J Tech Assess Health Care.* **9(1):** 26–36.

14 Torrance GW, Blacker D, Detsky A *et al.* (1996) Creating guidelines for economic evaluations in pharmaceuticals. *Pharmacoeconomics.* **9(6):** 553–9.

15 Coast J (1999) The appropriate uses of qualitative methods in health economics. *Health Economics.* **8:** 345–53.

16 Scott A, Currie N and Donaldson C (1998) Evaluating innovation in general practice: a pragmatic framework using programme budgeting and marginal analysis. *Fam Pract.* **15(3):** 216–22.

CHAPTER 18

Programme budgeting and marginal analysis: a pragmatic approach to economic evaluation

Ruth McDonald

Programme budgeting and marginal analysis (PBMA) is an attempt to incorporate some fundamental economic principles into a pragmatic framework that is accessible at grassroots level. Although in theory it is an attractive development, in practice it has found little application and there remain a number of barriers to its implementation.

Key points
- PBMA recognises that decision makers are not starting with a blank sheet of paper.
- The approach involves examining the existing allocation of resources in a particular programme and examining alternative ways of allocating those resources.
- In most cases the exercise aims to be resource neutral, but if new money is available it can help to identify where these resources can best be directed.
- It emphasises local cost and activity data, available evidence of effectiveness and value judgements of relevant stakeholders.

Chapter sections
- Introduction
- The two elements of PBMA – the programme budget and the marginal analysis
- The stages of programme budgeting and marginal analysis
- Getting PBMA into practice
- Conclusion

Introduction

Economic evaluation is underpinned by the 'rational' model of decision making. Chapter 17 has defined this model and the shortcomings of applying it to the complex environment of healthcare. However, decisions about resource allocation have to be made somehow. Some health policy commentators have suggested that given conflicting values, resource allocation must always be a process of debate.[1] This debate cannot always be resolved by an appeal to science or the refinement of 'rational' decision-making tools. What is important, it is argued, is that we ensure the debate will not be dominated by one particular interest. Historically, this has been the medical profession.

Health economists recognise that values conflict. For some, the response to a world in which values and goals conflict has been to roll up their sleeves and make the best of it. Programme budgeting and marginal analysis (PBMA) is a tool developed by economists to provide a framework for decision makers to incorporate evidence of effectiveness and cost effectiveness, as well as other criteria such as equity of access. PBMA recognises that decision makers are not starting with a blank sheet of paper to design ideal solutions. Hence, it involves examining the existing allocation of resources to a programme and examining alternative (usually resource neutral) ways of allocating those resources.

The two elements of PBMA – the programme budget and the marginal analysis

Programme budgeting (PB) and marginal analysis (MA) are two different, but linked, activities. The basic premise of PB is that it is important to understand how resources are currently spent before thinking about ways of changing this pattern of resource use. The premise underlying MA is that to have more of some services it is necessary to have less of others or, if growth monies are available, that some projects will be funded while others will not.

MA asks two questions.

- If additional resources were allocated to this programme how best could these be deployed to ensure the greatest possible increase in benefit?
- If resources for the programme are reduced, how best should these cuts be made to ensure the minimum loss of benefit from the programme?

PBMA combines these two elements and offers a framework that emphasises:

- use of local cost and activity data
- the availability of evidence on effectiveness
- an appreciation that many decisions are still based on value judgements, but the important thing is to be as open as possible about such judgements.

PBMA starts from the existing services and examines marginal changes in those services rather than starting with a blank piece of paper and attempting to allocate resources in some hypothetical fashion (Box 18.1).

Box 18.1:   An example of PBMA

To illustrate how PBMA would work in practice let's look at the example of a PCG that wants to improve services for people with coronary heart disease (CHD). The PCG doesn't have any more to spend, but has decided to use PBMA to investigate whether existing resources can be used to better effect.

   PBMA is a highly participative process. The PCG will need to establish a group of stakeholders to investigate the allocation of CHD resources. They will need to consider who should be involved, balancing the need for wide participation with manageable numbers at meetings. Having established a PBMA working group, criteria for decision making need to be identified. These might include effectiveness, waiting list targets and a preference for treating severe conditions. It may be that these criteria conflict. For example, somebody with a severe condition may benefit less from treatment (i.e. the effectiveness may be lower) than a less severely ill patient. It may be necessary, therefore, to weight criteria.

   The five-stage process is as follows:

- Step 1 – CHD has been identified as the programme area of interest.
- Step 2 – The PCG needs to identify all activity in primary, secondary and tertiary care. This will entail identifying items like drugs prescribed and GP consultations, emergency admissions to hospital with chest pain, outpatient appointments, tertiary investigations, surgery and invasive procedures, cardiac rehabilitation etc. In addition, the cost of all this activity should be identified using local cost data. The PCG might also choose to look beyond this at the impact on social services.
- Step 3 – Generate a list of candidates for service reduction and expansion. For example, by expanding the 'same day' chest pain clinic emergency admissions might be prevented; GPs could change to a more

cost effective first-line drug to reduce cholesterol; increasing cardiac rehabilitation services could reduce the incidence of future infarcts.

- Step 4 – Costs and benefits are assessed for each option. Benefits are assessed according to the criteria (values) agreed by stakeholders earlier.
- Step 5 – Recommendations for service changes. Thought will need to be given to the way in which these can be implemented. For example, if these entail purchasing fewer surgical procedures, this can be achieved through the contracting process. If GPs are to prescribe more cost effective drugs, how will this be delivered?

The stages of programme budgeting and marginal analysis

There are five stages in the PBMA framework:

- identification of a healthcare programme – usually disease based (e.g. cancers, coronary heart disease) or by client group (e.g. children, the elderly)
- production of a statement of expenditure and activity by subprogrammes – the programme budget (e.g. by primary, secondary and tertiary healthcare)
- generation of a list of candidate services for expansion and reduction
- measurement of the costs and benefits of proposed candidates for expansion and reduction (i.e. conduct marginal analysis)
- preparation of recommendations for purchasing.

Getting PBMA into practice

Advocates of PBMA claim that it is systematic, multidisciplinary and highly participative. In addition, it recognises that sacrifice is necessary and acknowledges the role of value judgements, while fostering a clear definition of objectives of health services. Critics point to disadvantages which include the significant amount of time, data, commitment and goodwill required from stakeholders and the difficulties associated with minimising vested interests. Lack of evidence of cost effectiveness and the difficulties in freeing up resources following small reductions in services may also serve to limit progress in practice.

Despite its attractions, the evidence suggests that PBMA has not had a great impact on resource allocation decisions at local level in the NHS. A recent international survey based study by Mitton and Donaldson[2] identified 78 cases where PBMA had been used in the last 25 years and found a 'positive impact' in 59% of studies. They noted that because their survey respondents were the authors of PBMA papers, the results may present a more favourable view of PBMA than would have been obtained by surveying health services personnel. Additionally, 'positive impact' is defined in terms of setting priorities or shifting resources, and the former may refer to the statement of priorities in policy documents, but with no resource shifts, the benefits obtained from these exercises are largely uncertain. A further cause for concern is that telephone calls, by the current author, to personnel in some of the NHS organisations (which the study suggest are using PBMA on an ongoing basis) revealed evidence to the contrary. These factors suggest caution in interpreting the results and that the study conclusions of widespread diffusion and positive impact may be overstated.

Appendix 2 reviews the PBMA studies that have been published and highlight a number of problems that occur even with the use of such a pragmatic approach to economic evaluation.

Problems with data collection and accuracy

Data collection in general was problematic. This relates to data on evidence as well as local costs and activity. For example, Twaddle and Walker identified a deficiency of their approach as 'applying flawed cost figures to activity data'.[3] Accurate cost data are not always available and collection of these data can prove challenging.

Complexity of health systems

Health systems are complex and dynamic. Changes in one service will have consequences for the rest of the system. Posnett and Street[4] criticise the 'essentially static' nature of many PBMA exercises. They argue for a model which identifies 'all relevant options prior to evaluation', an approach that places huge requirements on the information gathering and processing capabilities of individuals involved.

Conflict of values

A further potential problem concerns the reconciliation of conflicting value judgements or determining whose values were to count in the valuation process.

For example, Cohen's expert group identified criteria for use in their PBMA exercise, but abandoned attempts to weight these after failure to reach a consensus on the issue.[5] Part of the rationale for PBMA's 'expert group' phase is a recognition of the importance of obtaining consensus in relation to the value judgements, which inform the inputs to economic analysis. Such judgements include the extent to which the inclusion of inputs is seen as valid, the areas seen as legitimate for scrutiny, the valuation of intangibles (such as patient choice) and the weighting of criteria for decision making. However, while achieving consensus may allow economists to make progress when carrying out the analysis, it is important that those who are required to implement changes have some sense of ownership of the process.

Barriers to implementation

Only four of the eleven PBMA studies went beyond the production of results and reported the incorporation of proposals into contracts or strategy documents. None of the studies shed any light on how findings were (or were not) implemented! Two barriers to implementation were identified.

Practical problems with disinvestment

Lockett et al.[6] reported the failure to identify options for disinvestment, indicating that implementation would rely only on the receipt of any growth money. Other barriers to disinvestment include the inflexible NHS finance regimen and the inability to release cash where economic savings have been identified. This issue is raised in several of the PBMA studies that identified savings in hospitals but which, in practice, were not cash releasing. This may be because the health authorities concerned had weak legitimacy when it comes to disinvesting from existing services.

Problems with influencing the activity of service providers

Finally, there is a recognition that purchasers cannot command those who provide care. The move from hierarchical and top-down control to an emphasis on networks means that change must be negotiated.[7] Craig and colleagues[8] suggest that economic advice has made little progress because the purchaser/provider split obscures the fact that, in practice, resources are allocated by purchasers, hospital managers and doctors pursuing conflicting objectives which may not even be defined in the same terms. Changing clinical practice is difficult enough even when there is broad agreement on the benefits of doing so.

Implementation problems will be exacerbated if clinicians are unhappy with the choice of outcome or cost parameters in economic evaluation.

Conclusion

PBMA has been developed as a practical, participative and accessible framework that incorporates fundamental economic principles into decision making. However, the PBMA studies reviewed in this chapter raise many unanswered questions. The focus is largely on describing the PBMA methodology and its application. This is understandable as the aim appears to be to provide general information on methods to those considering the use of PBMA rather than a detailed consideration of how it can be actively used in practice. Available evidence suggests that it is possible to identify a range of factors at the construction, communication and implementation phases of health economic analyses that may limit the impact of studies on policy makers in practice. In certain areas (e.g. the NHS financial regimen) changes have been made which reduce these constraints, and the move towards unified budgets and changes in GP contracts will create incentives for PCTs and PCGs to utilise their resources more effectively.

The extent to which these changes will impact on the application of PBMA at local level is uncertain, but the evidence to date suggests that there is some way to go before this type of economic analysis enjoys widespread use among local decision makers. Experience to date shows that there remain many barriers to the development and implementation of this approach. Further research on the processes by which health economic analysis are commissioned, performed, communicated and implemented is required before firm conclusions can be drawn on how best to apply economic evaluation at grassroots level.

References

1   Klein R and Williams A (2000) Setting priorities: what is holding us back? In: A Coulter and C Ham (eds) *The Global Challenge of Health Care Rationing.* Open University Press, Buckingham.
2   Mitton C and Donaldson C (2001) Twenty five years of PBMA in the health sector. *J Health Serv Res Policy.* **6(4):** 239–48.
3   Twaddle S and Walker A (1996) Programme budgeting and marginal analysis: application within programmes to assist purchasing in Greater Glasgow Health Board. *Health Policy.* **33:** 91–105.

4   Posnett J and Street A (1996) Programme budgeting and marginal analysis: an approach in need of refinement. *J Health Serv Res Policy.* **1(3):** 147–53.
5   Cohen D (1994) Marginal analysis in practice: an alternative to needs assessment for contracting healthcare. *BMJ.* **309:** 781–5.
6   Lockett T, Raftery A and Richards J (1995) The strengths and limitations of programme budgeting. In: FR Honigsbaum, J Richards and T Lockett (eds) *Priority Setting in Action.* Radcliffe Medical Press, Oxford.
7   Rhodes R (1997) *Understanding Governance.* Open University Press, Buckingham.
8   Craig N, Parkin D and Gerard K (1995) Clearing the fog on the Tyne: programme budgeting in Newcastle and North Tyneside Health Authority. *Health Policy.* **33:** 107–25.

Section 5

Health economics and rationing

It is generally agreed by everyone, with the possible exception of government ministers, that not all citizens can receive the healthcare from which they could benefit. Difficult decisions are inevitable. The economic approach would choose interventions on the basis of their cost effectiveness, but international experience has demonstrated the difficulties of technical and explicit rationing frameworks. Unfortunately, there is no simple solution to the problem of who gets what and who goes without.

This section explores the complex inputs into the rationing agenda and the economic contribution to it. I start with an introduction to the healthcare rationing agenda outlining the options, but the inevitable conclusion seems to be that when price and the ability to pay are rejected as rationing devices, the whole thing is going to be a bit of a muddle.

In 1999, the National Institute for Clinical Excellence (NICE) was set up by government as part of its modernisation agenda. Its aim was to enable evidence of clinical and cost effectiveness to be integrated into decision making within the NHS and avoid the inequity of 'postcode' rationing. In Chapter 20, Rod Taylor, the former head of appraisals at NICE, and Rebecca Mears set NICE within the context of other international healthcare agencies and discuss the challenges of using economic evaluation in making decisions at national level.

An increasingly important input into the rationing debate is the view of the public. Unfortunately, what the public think, say and do are quite different matters. In Chapter 21, Mandy Ryan, Shelley Farrar and Caroline Reeves briefly outline how public opinion may be engaged before considering the technique of conjoint analysis as a method of quantifying this input.

What is efficient and what the public want may not be fair. In Chapter 22, Charles Normand discusses how a trade-off is often necessary between efficiency and a more equal or fairer distribution of services, illuminating the many difficulties in this area. But whatever the arguments about how we should ration, the agenda is underpinned by a legal framework that is often overlooked. In Chapter 23, Christopher Newdick explores the legal perspective, demonstrating the importance of historical precedent on the structure and process of decision making.

The complexities of the rationing agenda are most clearly illustrated by the recent case of beta interferon for the treatment of multiple sclerosis. NICE has ruled against its use on the grounds of limited cost effectiveness. Unable to face the harsh reality of rationing, the government has over-turned the scientific methodology that it expouses and launched an uncontrolled 'try it and see' approach across the NHS. At the time of going to press we await news as to whether new money will be available for this inter-esting manoeuvre or whether, as with most new drugs, savings will have to be made in other areas, where other patients will inevitably suffer or per-formance failure incurs punitive measures on decision makers. I explore the paradoxes of rationing in Chapter 30 by setting the whole area within an analytical framework provided by the theory of complex adap-tive systems.

CHAPTER 19

Healthcare rationing: an introduction

David Kernick

Although it is now generally agreed that not everyone can receive the healthcare from which they can benefit, international experience has confirmed that there is no simple solution to the problem of who gets what and who goes without. Health economists offer an input into the rationing process from the perspective of efficiency, but this does not always concur with what is equitable or with the views of the public.

Key points
- Rationing occurs when someone is denied a healthcare intervention that they need.
- Increasing demands on limited resources make rationing decisions inevitable.
- Rationing can be explicit or implicit.
- Explicit rationing can be undertaken by exclusion (i.e. the intervention is not available) or guidelines (i.e. the intervention is available but only to defined groups of patients).
- Health economists focus on developing explicit, technical and rational frameworks based on efficiency.
- There are other inputs into the decision-making process which include equity and public opinion.
- International experience suggests that rationing is inherently complex and there is no convergence to a common workable framework.

Chapter sections
- Introduction
- Rationing and equity
- Explicit or implicit rationing?
- Rationing – the international experience

- An alternative approach to rationing – managing need
- Conclusion

Introduction

The central economic problem for society is how to reconcile the desire for goods and services and the scarcity of resources with which they can be produced. Although the market provides an efficient distribution mechanism based on price and the ability to pay there are a number of fundamental problems applying this approach to healthcare. The most practical concern is that a market approach is unfair or inequitable. Central to the rationing agenda is the concept of needs and wants. Klein[1] contrasts the language of wants – what the patient thinks will benefit him or her (reflecting a market philosophy and consumer sovereignty) – with the language of the needs – what an agent sanctioned by society thinks will benefit the patient (reflecting paternalism from healthcare experts). In this analysis, rationing in the NHS amounts to a failure to meet expert determined need.

The traditional interpretation of rationing was a positive concept, donating a share or portion of a predetermined size to which each qualified recipient was entitled. More recently, rationing has become a metaphor with negative, prerogative overtones – scarcity, denial, withdrawal and inevitable suffering. Priority setting is used as a less prerogative term. The intervention is available but not accessible to all patients. Hope is not extinguished and the emphasis is on guidelines and protocols rather than definitive exclusions.

Perhaps the simplest solution to rationing is to simply deny that there is a problem and hope that it will go away. This appears to be the current mode favoured by government that still espouses a health service that is comprehensive, of high quality and freely available on the basis of need. A variation of the 'no problem' theme is the suggestion that the limits to demand are within the capacity of a properly resourced NHS and that the system contains the potential for efficiency gains which could release sufficient resources to match demand.[2] This argument has found little support but, undoubtedly, there is room for some efficiency gains, and healthcare spending is being increased.

Assuming that difficult decisions are inevitable, an alternative approach to the market model is to make decisions within a sociably negotiated framework. This can take two forms:

- distribution based on defined rules of entitlement – explicit rationing
- discretion of gatekeepers that determine access into the system (for example GPs) – implicit rationing.

Three basic principles of rationing have been defined:[3]

- to treat equals equally and with due dignity especially near death
- to meet people's needs for healthcare as efficiently as possible (imposing least sacrifice on others)
- to minimise inequalities in the lifetime health of the population.

Although most people would sign up for these laudable aims, applying them in practice is another matter.

Rationing can occur at a number of levels of the NHS, and there may be conflict between the perspectives of each level (Box 19.1). For example, clinicians have a primary obligation to do what is best for their patient, healthcare managers adopt a public health perspective and politicians attempt to balance the nation's resources fairly between competing sectors.

Box 19.1:   The five levels of rationing

Level 1   How much to allocate to the NHS in competition with other agencies, such as education, defence, housing?

Level 2   How much to allocate across sectors (e.g. mental health, cancer, ischaemic heart disease?)

Level 3   How much to allocate specific interventions within sectors (e.g. should multiple sclerosis be treated with drugs or physiotherapy?)

Level 4   How much to allocate interventions between different patients in the same group (e.g. which patients with raised cholesterol should be treated?)

Level 5   How much to invest in each patient once an intervention has been initiated (e.g. how low should cholesterol be lowered in treated patients?)

Rationing and equity

The NHS was built on the idea of social justice and remains explicitly committed to the principle of equity. However, things have changed little over the past 20 years since the Black report highlighted the social inequalities in health in the UK. There remain two major problems.

First, no one is really quite sure what equity means and there are a number of perspectives on what is 'fair', summarised in Box 19.2. The ethics of healthcare distribution is an area hedged with arguments and counterarguments without any convergence to a workable solution. Perhaps the most common interpretation is that people should receive healthcare on the basis of need and not who they are and those with greater need should receive preferential treatment.

Second, there is the inevitable conflict between equity and efficiency concerns. What is fair is not usually efficient and often leads to inconsistent judgements in healthcare policies. For example, the NHS policy on cervical cancer screening is directed at an efficient coverage through the use of financial incentives to GPs. We strive to attain our efficiency targets rather than focusing on those most disadvantaged who do not take up our offer of a smear test but who are most at risk. A recent review of the literature on economic evaluation[4] demonstrated a complete neglect of the equity dimension. The studies surveyed did not provide enough information for decision-makers to make their own judgements about the impact on various population groups affected by the policy under study.

Some health economists have tried to address these issues by developing an equity weighted QALY but there appear to be insurmountable theoretical and practical problems. Perhaps the best approach is to present information on the cost implications and benefits in different population groups. Decision makers can then apply their own values and trade-offs to the choices that have to be made taking into account national policy and local considerations.

Box 19.2:   Some approaches to what is fair

- People should receive healthcare in proportion to their contribution to society.
- Those who are older have had their fair innings and should receive less.
- Everyone should receive an equal proportion of healthcare resources.
- Available resources should be used to equalise the health of the population to some common level.
- Everyone should have equal access to care.
- Health resources should be directed at those who are most unwell (irrespective of how they would benefit).
- Health resources should be directed at those who are most unwell and who would benefit most.
- Health care resources should be distributed in such a way to maximise the benefit of society overall. (This is the approach of health economics based on utilitarianism. It could infer that those who are most unwell would receive no healthcare at all, as the advantaged groups in society may have a superior capacity to benefit).

Explicit or implicit rationing?

Views on rationing fall into three camps.

- The whole thing is so complex that the best approach is to muddle through and keep things out of the public eye as much as possible.
- Rationing should be explicit and based on technical frameworks that relate benefits of competing interventions to their costs.
- There is no simple answer to rationing but decision making must be open and transparent.

Historically (Box 19.3), decision making in the NHS has been 'a combination of guidelines, exhortation and obfuscation, leaving it largely to the coal face workers to jiggle a quart of services from a pint pot of resources'.[6] Stakeholders were happy to acquiesce to this system where doctors made implicit rationing decisions without challenge.

Over the last decade the call to make rationing more explicit has been driven by a number of factors:

- a more educated and informed consumer
- a concern that decision making may be influenced by political and professional interests rather than those of patients
- implicit rationing may not represent effective or efficient use of resources
- availability of interventions varies across the country
- the intrinsic benefits of honesty and openness in a democratic society.

Not everyone is in favour of explicit rationing and there is no evidence that it will improve the well being of society as a whole. Some commentators argue that rationing is an unavoidable messy affair and that there are dangers in spurious

---

Box 19.3: Five historical rationing mechanisms[5]

- Deterrent – the demands for healthcare are obstructed (e.g. prescription and dental charges, inconvenient location of services)
- Delay – waiting lists modulate excess demands
- Deflection – GPs deflect demand from secondary care and may shift it into other sectors and budgets
- Dilution – for example, fewer tests, cheaper drugs
- Denial – an arbitrary range of services is denied to patients which results in postcode rationing (e.g. cosmetic surgery, reversal of sterilisation, infertility treatment)

and risky rational approaches. For example, Machanic[7] has argued that discretional rationing can respond more flexibly and sensitively to the heterogeneity of patients, doctors and their treatments. The traditional elements of judgement and intuition act in the individual patient's interest unlike the rigid alternative of a superficial assessment of equity/efficiency trade-offs. Butler[5] argues that a sensitive and intelligent kind of muddling through seems to accord with the reality of how things are done at the coal face and argues that the discourses about what is right and what is feasible must keep in step with each other.

The evidence suggests that although citizens wish to be consulted, they do not want to make rationing decisions directly, and view doctors as the most appropriate group to take these decisions on behalf of society.[8] This desire of citizens to employ an agent to make societal rationing decisions is based on two factors. First, a lack of knowledge, objectivity and consistency. Empirical work has suggested that citizens are unable to reach agreement about general principles and that their preferences can change with time.[9,10] Second, a potential for distress as a result of an involvement in the denial of care. Being confronted with the harsh reality of rationing can lead to disutility for both decisions makers and patients.[11]

Rationing – the international experience

A number of explicit rationing frameworks have been tried, notably in Oregon, the Netherlands, New Zealand and Sweden. The evidence to date suggests that rationing is inherently complex and not amenable to a quick fix. Two key approaches have been identified – rationing services by exclusion (exclusion of whole categories of services) and establishing priorities using guidelines (offering a broad range of interventions but limiting access to defined groups). A universal theme has been the involvement of the public at all stages of the process.

Despite moves towards making resource decisions using technical frameworks in a manner that is both fair and explicit, international experience demonstrates that rationing is messy and there appears to be no convergence to a common workable solution or an explicit framework which is acceptable both publicly and politically.[12] Value judgements, estimates and gut feelings remain the predominant determinates of outcome.[13] Each country may need to find its own solutions reflecting its own circumstances and history, but a common theme seems to be that decisions are made openly and not behind closed doors.

In the UK, the National Institute for Clinical Excellence (NICE) has been established to make recommendations at a national level. How this body operates and the problems that it has encountered are considered in Chapter 20.

An alternative approach to rationing – managing need

A current approach to health service pressure is demand management – modulating what the patient wants or feels will do him/her good. An alternative solution would be to manage need – what the medical/industrial complex thinks would benefit a patient. Chapter 2 has highlighted the problem of supplier induced demands. The very people who decide what we need are the ones who develop, produce and supply those services.

In 1966, Enoch Powell, the Minister of Health, noted that 'every advance in medical science creates new needs that did not exist until the means of meeting them came into existence or into the realms of the possible'. Do we actually want the outpourings of the modern medical machine that are the cause of the rationing dilemma?

Although medical science has undoubtedly had some spectacular successes, the contribution of personal medical interventions has for some time been recognised as tertiary when compared to behavioural and environmental factors.[14] Of the 30-year increase in life expectancy that has occurred in the twentieth century, medical interventions have contributed only 5 years[15] and the best estimates are that health services influence only 10% of the usual indices for measuring health. Over the past 20 years nearly all of these extra years have been marked by the presence of limiting long-term illness. Expectancy of years free from limiting long-term illness increased by just 0.8 years for men and 0.1 years for women.[16] Perhaps of greater concern is the increase in self-reported ill health in all age groups over the past 30 years.[17]

Are we doing better but feeling worse? It is interesting to note that the two decades in the twentieth century that have seen the biggest improvement in life expectancy were 1910–1919 and 1940–1949 (other than for combatants), offering an important clue to the important relationship between health and social cohesion.[18] Is the healthcare industry creating a supplier-induced need and inducing an unnecessary rationing agenda, consuming resources that could provide greater marginal benefit in health if shifted elsewhere?

Conclusion

Health economists have focused on developing explicit, technical and rational frameworks based on efficiency to facilitate rationing choices, and economic evaluation is a theme which runs throughout this book. Undoubtedly, there are a number of health economists who dream of a health service where resource decisions are made using equity-weighted quality adjusted life years, but this denies the constraints and contingencies of the real world.

What is efficient may not be what is fair or just, and there are a number of ethical philosophies that seek to inform healthcare rationing. Unfortunately, this area is hedged with constraints, intermediate positions, arguments and counter arguments. Most theoretical ethical models are either unworkable or have not been utilised to any extent in practice. Perhaps the only theme on which there is broad agreement is the importance of involving the public in rationing decisions. However, the public may not deliver a just or efficient solution even if they are ready to enter the rationing arena.

There remain two interesting features of the healthcare rationing agenda. First, it generates a disproportional level of debate compared with other public sectors such as education, housing and environment that may offer a greater contribution towards health gain. Second, the voluminous literature in the area reflects a preoccupation with explicitness and transparency at the expense of the development of workable solutions.

It does seem that, when price and the ability to pay are rejected as a mechanism to distribute limited resources, we can be sure that there will be no easy answers to who gets what and who goes without. If a workable solution were available, it would be likely that someone would have found it by now.

References

1   Kline R (1995) *The New Politics of the NHS*. Longman, Harlow.
2   Frankel S, Ebrahim S and Davey-Smith G (2000) The limits to demand for healthcare. *BMJ*. **321**: 40–5.
3   Williams A, Hutton J and Maynard A (2000) A NICE challenge for health economists. *Health Economics*. **9**: 89–93.
4   Sassi F, Archard I and LeGrand J (2001) Equity and economic evaluation of healthcare. *Health Technol Assess*. **5(3)**.
5   Hunter D (1997) *Desperately Seeking Solutions*. Longman, London.
6   Butler J (1999) *The Ethics of Healthcare Rationing*. Cassell, London.
7   Machanic D (1995) Dilemmas in rationing healthcare services: the case for implicit rationing. *BMJ*. **310**: 1655–9.
8   Kneeshaw J (1997) What does the public think about rationing? A review of the evidence. In: B New (ed) *Rationing Talk and Action in Healthcare*. BMJ Publishing, London.
9   Cuadras-Morato X and Pinto-Prades J (2001) Equity considerations in health care: the relevance of claims. *Health Economics*. **10**: 187–205.
10 Shiell A, Seymour J, Hawe P *et al.* (2000) Are preferences over health states complete? *Health Economics*. **9**: 47–55.
11 Coast J (1997) Rationing within the NHS should be explicit. The case against. *BMJ*. **314**: 118–22.

12 World Health Organization (1996) *European Healthcare Reforms: analysis and current strategies*. World Health Organization Regional Office for Europe, Copenhagen.
13 Honigsbaum F, Richards J and Lockett T (1995) *Priority Setting and Action: purchasing dilemmas*. Radcliffe Medical Press, Oxford.
14 McKeown T (1979) *The Role of Medicine*. Blackwell, Oxford.
15 Bunker J and Frazier F (1994) Improving health measurement. Effects of health and medical care. *Milbank Quarterly*. **72(2):** 225–58.
16 Bevington A and Darton R (1996) *Health Life Expectancy in England and Wales: Recent Evidence*. PSSRU Discussion Paper 1205. University of Canterbury, Canterbury.
17 *General Household Survey 1999* (2000) HMSO, London.
18 Sen A (1999) *Development as Freedom*. Knopf, New York.

CHAPTER 20

Making decisions at a national level: a NICE experience?

Rod Taylor and Rebecca Mears

The National Institute for Clinical Excellence (NICE) was established in 1999 to enable evidence of clinical and cost effectiveness to be integrated into decision making within the NHS. This chapter describes the structure and function of NICE in context with other international healthcare agencies, and discusses the challenges of using economic evaluation in making decisions at a national level.

Key points
- NICE is a new organisation tasked with advising the health service on how it should use new drugs and other healthcare interventions based on a rigorous assessment of cost effectiveness.
- Although there a number of other national agencies in other countries who undertake economic evaluations, only a very small number have a mandate for issuing policy at a national level.
- Using evidence of cost effectiveness in national policy making has a number of challenges in both the process of assessment and implementation of findings.

Chapter sections
- Introduction
- National decision making – the international picture
- NICE – a UK model of national decision making
- The challenges of national decision making
- Consistency of decision making
- Conclusion

Introduction

Decision making in primary care has traditionally focused on individual patient decisions made at the level of the practitioner. The recent development of primary care groups/trusts (PCG/T) across the NHS will result in many decisions about the availability of particular therapies and healthcare services now being made at a population level. However, due to the rise in both healthcare costs and demand, many countries have begun to implement a national system of decision making which includes not only the three requirements of quality, safety and efficacy but in addition, the consideration of cost effectiveness – the so-called 'fourth hurdle'.

The government paper *A First Class Service*[1] defined the aims of the National Institute for Clinical Excellence (NICE) which was set up in April 1999 to 'enable evidence of clinical and cost effectiveness to be integrated to inform a national judgement on the value of a treatment(s) relative to alternative uses of the resources' and thereby provide 'guidance on whether a treatment (new or existing) can be recommended for routine use in the NHS (in England and Wales)'. A similar framework is being established in Scotland. Figure 20.1 sets

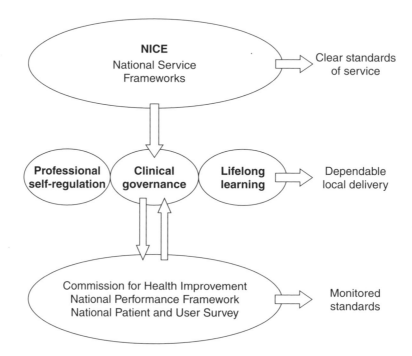

Figure 20.1: NICE in context. Setting, delivering and monitoring standards.

Box 20.1: Some NICE terminology

Health technology – any method used by those working in health services to promote health, screen, diagnose and treat disease and improve rehabilitation and long-term care.

Health technology assessment – considers the effectiveness, appropriateness, cost and broader implications of technologies using both primary research and systematic review. It seeks to meet the information needs of those who manage and provide care.

A systematic review – a review of the evidence on a clearly formulated question that uses systematic and explicit methods to identify, select and critically appraise relevant primary research, and to extract and analyse data from the studies that are included in the review.

Mandatory recommendations – advice to healthcare professionals that is obligatory.

Advisory recommendations – advice to healthcare professionals that is guidance and therefore whose implementation involves clinical judgement.

---

out how NICE will provide national standards with local responsibility for their delivery, backed with a consistent monitoring processes such as that provided by the Commission for Health Improvement (CHI).

This chapter will describe the structure and function of NICE in the context of other international healthcare agencies, illustrate its role with reference to one of its recent decisions directly influencing primary care and discuss some of the current challenges of using economic evaluations in making decisions at a national level. Some NICE terminology is provided in Box 20.1.

National decision making – the international picture

Health technology assessment (HTA) has become an accepted approach to assisting decision makers at national and subnational levels to decide whether or not to implement technologies or treatments. Many countries have now established agencies tasked with this remit. The International Society for Technology Assessment in Health Care (ISTAHC) and the International Network of

Agencies for Heath Technology Assessment (INAHTA) are organisations specifically concerned with promoting an international network of HTA agencies.[2,3]

A recent survey of HTA agencies from across Europe,[4] the Americas and Australasia examined the role of economic evaluation in national decision making. Of the 97 agencies surveyed, 52 (54%) responded. Although virtually all agencies (90%) included assessment of clinical effectiveness, only 76% undertook some form of economic assessment. All of these reported incorporating cost effectiveness analysis, and 56% of respondents reported using cost utility and/or cost benefit analysis as part of their normal practice.

The national responsibility of these agencies included decisions on regulation, reimbursement, quality assurance, healthcare education and training. In the majority of cases, input into national decision making was advisory rather than mandatory. The results of this international review indicate the importance of both clinical and cost effectiveness evidence to national healthcare decision-making systems when new treatments are being considered. However, there are other important inputs into the decision-making process which include elements such as affordability, safety and the views of key stakeholders and expert groups.

NICE – a UK model of national decision making

What does NICE do?

NICE's mandate includes two principal areas of national decision-making responsibility:

- clinical guidelines programme (i.e. development of national guidance focusing on an area of disease management)
- technology appraisals programme (i.e. national guidance on the use of specific healthcare technologies).

The technologies and guidelines that have been either referred to NICE or published to date by NICE are listed in Tables 20.1 and 20.2. The technology appraisal programme represents NICE's main output of national guidance to date and has also undergone the most development and received the most public and media attention. The remainder of this section will therefore, focus on the appraisal process.

Table 20.1:   Clinical guidelines referred by the Department of Health and the National Assembly of Wales to NICE (as of April 2001)

Non-insulin dependent diabetes
Early pharmacological management of schizophrenia
Pressure sores prevention (published April 2001)
Head and neck cancer
Haematological malignancies
Skin cancer
Foetal monitoring
Peptic ulcer and dyspepsia
Multiple sclerosis
Management of depression in the community
Induction of labour
Management of myocardial infarction in primary care
Hypertension
Routine preoperative investigations

Table 20.2:   Technology appraisals published by NICE (as of April 2001)

Relenza (zanamivir) for influenza
Removal of wisdom teeth
Selection of prostheses for primary total hip replacement
Taxanes for ovarian cancer
Coronary artery stents for ischaemic heart disease
Liquid-based cytology for cervical screening
Taxanes for breast cancer
Proton pump inhibitors in the treatment of dyspepsia
Hearing aid technology
Glitazones for type II diabetes mellitus
Inhaler systems (devices) for children under the age of 5 years with chronic asthma
Ribavarin/interferon-alpha for hepatitis C
Methylphenidate for attention deficit hyperactivity disorder
GP IIb/IIIa inhibitors for acute coronary syndromes
Wound care
Implantable cardioverter defibrillators for cardiac arrhythmias
Drugs for Alzheimer's disease
Riluzole for motor disease
Autologous cartilage transplantation
Laproscopic surgery for colorectal cancer and inguinal hernias
Orilstat for obesity

Which technologies are assessed?

Unlike Australia, where decisions are made about the availability of all new drugs based on cost effectiveness, only a small proportion of possible healthcare technologies are referred to NICE. The Department of Health and the National Assembly for Wales currently undertake responsibility for identification, selection and referral of technologies to NICE. This selection is based on one or more of the following criteria.

- Is the technology likely to result in a significant health benefit taken across the NHS as a whole if given to all patients for whom it is indicated?
- Is the technology likely to result in a significant impact on other health-related government policies (e.g. reduction in health inequalities)?
- Is the technology likely to have a significant impact on NHS resources (financial or other) if given to all patients for whom it is indicated?

Only a relatively small proportion of all new therapies relevant to primary care practitioners will ever be subject to national guidance by NICE. Therefore, despite the growing amount of national guidance such as that of NICE and the National Service Frameworks, there remains a need for 'local decision making' on those technologies not covered by such national advice.

The process of assessment

In common with other international agencies, health technology assessment underpins NICE's appraisal of a technology. The HTA reports produced by NICE are each undertaken over a period of approximately 6 months by a panel of UK university research units commissioned through the NHS R&D HTA Programme. These reports include a detailed systematic review of clinical and cost effectiveness of the technology using Cochrane-based methods. In addition, reports include a review of a submission by the manufacturer of each technology. Industry submissions often include additional data, such as unpublished clinical trials and economic modelling.

Making the decision

The specific responsibility for this decision making falls upon the NICE Appraisal Committee – a standing committee of independent experts drawn from the health professions, patient-focused organisations, health service researchers, healthcare managers and the pharmaceutical industry. The membership is composed of individuals who can take both a specific and wider view of the evidence presented to them, although topic specific experts can be coopted. The evidence considered by the committee includes the HTA report and submissions

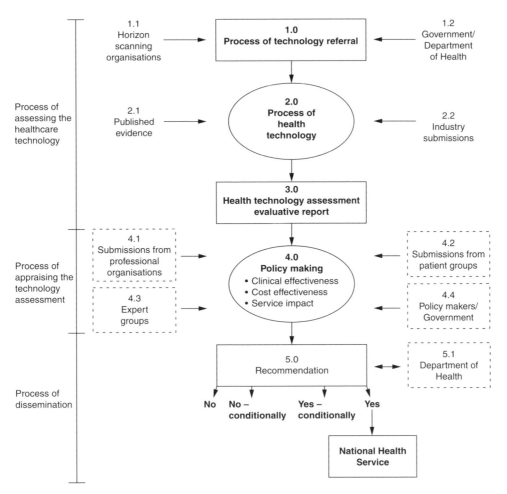

Figure 20.2:   Framework of the healthcare decision-making process undertaken by NICE within its technology appraisal programme.

invited from key stakeholders that include manufacturers, national professional groups and patient-advocate groups. NICE accepts and formally issues this guidance to the NHS in England and Wales following consultation with these key stakeholders (Figure 20.2).

Acting on the decision

The aim of NICE is to assess a predetermined number of healthcare technologies annually and as a result, formulate and issue national guidance. Unlike most international HTA agencies, NICE has a formal mandate for national policy making. However, the status of NICE's guidance, unlike drug regulation authorities, is advisory rather that mandatory. Its decisions do not represent direction to healthcare professionals, and implementation of this advice involves clinical judgement. There remains uncertainty over the extent to which NICE's advice is adopted. Nevertheless it is important to remember that one role of the Commission for Health Improvement is to audit the action taken by health authorities and PCG/Ts on NICE and other national guidance.

The challenges of national decision making

The Relenza case study

Box 20.2 shows a case study of the drug Relenza. A number of issues regarding national decision making arise from this study.

The changing face of evidence

The Relenza study highlights that the evidence base of both clinical and cost effectiveness of new technology is often an evolving one. An important trial using Relenza in 'high-risk' groups was still being undertaken by the manufacturer during NICE's first appraisal in 1999. The potential risks of such early assessment of healthcare technologies are further considered below.

Guidance – mandatory or advisory

The output of the NICE decision-making process, as with most other international HTA agencies, is guidance that is not mandatory. For example, a number of PCG/Ts were 'not happy' with NICE's revised decision to recommend Relenza for high-risk individuals and threatened not to implement the guidance.[5]

Risks of early assessment

There is pressure for national decision makers to assess the cost effectiveness of a health technology as early as possible (i.e. at or just after the point of licensing). The strength of early assessment is to promote the more rapid diffusion of cost effective technologies into practice and inhibit the inappropriate diffusion of those technologies that are not cost effective. However, this has to be

Box 20.2:   Relenza – a NICE case study

Relenza (zanamivir) was the first of a new generation of antiviral agents licensed in the UK in 1999 as a prescription only treatment for patients who present with influenza-like symptoms. At £24 per 5-day course, Relenza represented a new health technology for a potentially self-limiting illness but with significant costs implications to the NHS. Relenza was referred to NICE for appraisal, first in 1999 and then again in 2000 .

This case study is interesting in that there was a change in the decision made by NICE regarding its recommendation. In October 1999, NICE issued guidance recommending 'that health professionals should not pre-scribe Relenza'. In November 2000, NICE revised its decision, issuing the guidance that Relenza should be 'recommended when influenza is circu-lating in the community ... for the treatment of high-risk individuals'. Some of the underlying reasons for this change in decision, taken from NICE guidance, are summarised below.

Summary of NICE's appraisal of Relenza

	First appraisal October 1999	*Second appraisal November 2000*
Focus of appraisal	Treatment of influenza across all groups	Treatment of influenza in 'high-risk' patients only
The evidence base	3 randomised controlled trials $n = 1167$ individuals (14% high risk)	As before plus a 'high-risk' trial. 800 patients with chest disease
Clinical effectiveness	Median reduction in time to alleviation of symptoms of 1 day (95% CI: 0.5–1.5 days)	Reduction in absolute risk of complications requiring antibiotics
Cost effectiveness	None calculated	£9300 to £31,500 per quality adjusted life year
Budget impact for NHS England and Wales	£9.9 to £15 million	£2.3 to £11.7 million

balanced with the potential risk of early assessment which is that the evidence base for the technology is unlikely to be fully developed and, therefore, there is the risk of getting the decision wrong! Early assessment may result in effective innovations being discarded or ineffective ones being accepted. As the Relenza example illustrates, although there may be an imperative for early assessment there is also a need for decision makers to be able to revisit a technology once the evidence base has matured.

Cost effectiveness or affordability?

Decision makers with scare resources are not only concerned with the cost effectiveness of health technologies but with the potential budgetary impact that making new technologies available could have. Cost effectiveness does not infer affordability and in many cases the latter may be more important. Consider the example shown in Table 20.3 where a primary care trust (PCT) is deciding to implement one of two possible technologies.

Table 20.3:   The hypothetical cost effectiveness and budget impact for two technologies

Intervention	Incremental cost per QALY (cost effectiveness)	Net cost of intervention treatment course	Number of patients requiring therapy	Total budget impact
A	£45,000	£1500	10	£15,000
B	£19,000	£4000	2500	£1,000,000

On the basis of cost effectiveness, the PCT may favour technology B. However, from the perspective of affordability the decision may be reversed because technology A is used to treat a relatively rare condition and overall has a more favourable budgetary impact.

The relative role of cost effectiveness and budgetary impact to decision making remains a largely unexplored area. At present, the role of NICE is to make its national decisions on the basis of cost effectiveness rather than affordability. However, decision makers who are faced with implementing national agency recommendations with limited budgets must consider both. Affordability was raised as an issue following the NICE guidance on using Relenza in high-risk patients.[5]

Consistency of decision making

Decisions across healthcare sectors (e.g. a new cardiovascular treatment versus a new cancer therapy) require a common metric so that different technologies can be directly compared. Cost utility analysis and the resultant cost per QALY has the benefit of providing decision makers with an outcome that allows them to make explicit the trade-off in making decisions across healthcare sectors. However, it must be recognised that there remains a lack of consensus in the derivation and utilisation of the QALY.

When agencies are using cost utility studies across sequential decisions, consistency is required. One approach is to define a maximum threshold of willingness to pay for each QALY, and all technologies with a cost per QALY in excess of this threshold are rejected. However, there is currently no consensus on the value of this maximum cost per QALY threshold, and issues remain as to how decision makers would use this approach. For example, if a new treatment represents the only clinically effective intervention in a therapeutic area, should national decision makers set their threshold cost higher? How do decision makers decide on new technologies where a cost per QALY may either not yet be available or inappropriate? For example, in the case of Relenza, is a cost per QALY an appropriate measure for an acute self-limiting illness?

Conclusion

In the current climate of increasing healthcare demand and limited resources, national decision makers need to consider clinical cost effectiveness when deciding on whether to implement new treatments into routine clinical practice. Many countries have developed national HTA agencies to undertake assessment of the cost effectiveness of new treatments in order to inform such decisions. NICE, however, is currently only one of relatively few international 'fourth hurdle' agencies with a formal mandate for the issuance of national guidance. Nevertheless, for those in primary care who are faced with implementation of NICE guidance there remain some fundamental issues, which are reviewed in this chapter.

One of the main reasons that NICE was established was to abolish postcode prescribing. Ironically, it may be that NICE guidance may now only be shifting the problem from the level of postcodes to individual PCG/T's and hospital trusts. Organisations such as the Commission for Health Improvement will certainly play a key role in monitoring the adherence to national guidance in the future. We watch with interest!

References

1   Department of Health (1997) *A First Class Service: quality in the new NHS*. NHS Executive, Leeds.

2   International Society for Technology Assessment in Health Care website address: http://www.istahc.org/

3   International Network of Agencies for Heath Technology Assessment website address: http://www.inahta.org/

4   Mears R, Taylor R, Littlejohns P and Dillon A (2000) *Review of International Health Technology Assessment (IHTA)*. Final Report, National Institute for Clinical Excellence, June 2000. http://www.nice.org/

5   Powell M (2001) Latest decision on zanamivir will not end postcode prescribing (Letter). *BMJ*. **322**: 489.

CHAPTER 21

Obtaining the views of the public: using conjoint analysis studies when eliciting preferences in healthcare

Mandy Ryan, Shelley Farrar and Caroline Reeves

A number of approaches have been developed to obtain the views of patients and the public on how resources should be allocated. Economic techniques for eliciting public preferences all include the notion of sacrifice or trading. This chapter briefly reviews the methods available and in particular the role of conjoint analysis.

Key points
- NHS decision makers need to have information on patient and public views about healthcare in order to be good agents.
- Conjoint analysis is a rigorous method for eliciting patient and public preferences.
- It allows estimation of the relative importance of different aspects of care, the trade-offs between these aspects, and the total satisfaction or utility that respondents derive from healthcare.
- While further applications of conjoint analysis are encouraged, methodological issues need addressing.

Chapter sections
- **Introduction**
- **Conjoint analysis**
- **An application in general practice**
- **Conclusion**

Introduction

It has always been the role of decision makers in the NHS to act on behalf of the less informed and less empowered general public. To be effective in this agency role, the decision maker requires information on the needs, demands and wants of society. Traditionally, focus has been on the needs of the population which have been measured by clinicians and epidemiologists. Giving patients and the general public a role in decision making on the allocation of resources in the NHS, whether it is at the level of setting national or local priorities or inputting into the configuration of local healthcare services, is a relatively new concept. The NHS reforms of the 1990s introduced the concept of consumerism into healthcare and it has remained there in so far as there is a responsibility to take into account local wants as well as needs in the provision of services.[1-6] In principle, the elicitation of patient/community views represents a step forward in terms of enhancing benefits from the provision of healthcare. However, for the exercise to be worthwhile, the information obtained must be applicable and scientifically defensible.[7]

Numerous methods have been used to obtain the views of consumers. These are shown in Table 21.1. Ryan *et al.*[8] provide information on these techniques.

Economic techniques for eliciting public preferences all include the notion of sacrifice or trading. Such techniques are based on the assumption that something is only of value if an individual is willing to give something up for it. Given the limited budget in healthcare, devoting more resources to improve one aspect of a service means taking resources away from another aspect (i.e. there is a sacrifice of benefit or an opportunity cost – where opportunity cost is defined as the benefits foregone from not using resources in their next

Table 21.1:　Methods of eliciting public preferences for health care (see Ryan *et al.* www. ncchta.org)

Quantitative techniques	Qualitative techniques
Non trade-off methods	• Interviews
• Ranking technique	• Case study analysis
• Rating techniques (e.g. visual analogue scale)	• Delphi technique
• Likert scale	• Focus groups
• Alternative choice based techniques	• Consensus panels
	• Citizens jury
Trade-off methods	• Public meeting
• Standard gamble	
• Time trade-off	
• Willingness to pay	
• Conjoint analysis	

best alternative use). For example, the opportunity cost of introducing a patient healthcare card (see later in this chapter) is the benefit that would have accrued had the resources been spent on improving other aspects of general practice (e.g. reducing waiting time between an appointment and seeing the doctor; reducing waiting time in surgery; giving patients choice over the doctor they see). Given limited resources, and the fact that individuals would prefer improvements in all aspects of care, choices have to be made. In these circumstances the relevant policy questions are then what are the relative weights of the important dimensions of benefits, how do individuals trade-off these dimensions, and, given these trade-offs, what is the optimal way to provide a service?

Techniques developed in health economics to elicit user views explicitly address these questions. The three main methods used have been standard gamble (SG), time trade-off (TTO) and willingness to pay (WTP).[8] SG embodies the notion of sacrifice by asking individuals to sacrifice certainty, TTO asks individuals to trade time and WTP asks individuals to trade money. SG and TTO have been developed within the quality adjusted life year (QALY) paradigm which assumes that only health outcomes are important. As such, satisfaction or utility has become synonymous with health outcomes. Such utility measures are inappropriate for valuing non-health outcomes (e.g. information) and process attributes (waiting time, choice), where utility is defined as broader than health outcomes. While WTP can take account of non-health outcomes and process attributes, many individuals object to this technique because of a political objection to paying for healthcare, and because of its relationship to ability to pay. Conjoint analysis has been identified as a potential instrument that could overcome the limitations of QALYs and WTP.

This chapter demonstrates how conjoint analysis can be a useful technique for eliciting patient and public preferences. The next section gives some background to the technique and presents the steps involved in undertaking a conjoint analysis exercise. Following this, an example is drawn from primary care to demonstrate the applicability of the instrument.

Conjoint analysis

Conjoint analysis was developed in mathematical psychology[9,10] and has been widely used in marketing,[11] transport economics[12] and more recently environmental economics.[13] The technique is gaining widespread use in healthcare and has been applied successfully in a wide range of areas including: eliciting patient/community preferences in the delivery of health services; establishing consultants' preferences in priority setting; developing outcome measures; determining optimal treatments for patients; evaluating alternatives within randomised controlled trials; and establishing patient preferences in the doctor–patient relationship.[8,14–23]

Data are collected in conjoint analysis studies by asking respondents, in a questionnaire format, to rank, rate or select their preferred choices from a number of services and/or treatments. These services or treatments are described in terms of a number of predetermined characteristics (or attributes) considered important for that service. The process of data collection and analysis can be divided into five stages.

Stage 1: Identifying the characteristics

This can be done by various methods. If a policy question is being addressed, the characteristics will be predefined. For example, in a study concerned with the value of reducing waiting time for elective surgery on the Isle of Wight the attributes in the study were defined as travel costs, location of treatment and waiting time.[21] Similarly, in a study concerned with the optimal location of an orthodontic clinic, the attributes were defined as location of first appointment, location of second appointment and waiting time.[24] For use alongside a randomised controlled trial, the different outcome measures and process characteristics of the arms of the trial may define the characteristics. For example, in a study concerned with the optimal management of miscarriage, the attributes, which included level of pain, time in hospital receiving treatment, time taken to return to normal activities and complications, were taken directly from the results of a randomised, controlled trial.[23] Where the characteristics are not predefined, literature reviews or qualitative research methods may be used. A study concerned with the preferences of South Australians for public hospital services used a series of focus groups to determine the most important attributes in choice of hospital services.[25]

Stage 2: Assigning levels to the characteristics

Each characteristic is given levels. These may be cardinal (e.g. waiting time where 2 weeks is twice as long as 1 week), ordinal (e.g. while 'severe pain' is worse than 'moderate pain', we do not know by how much) or categorical (e.g. where there is no natural ordering for specialist nurse, general practitioner or consultant). The levels must be plausible and actionable thus encouraging respondents to take the exercise seriously. Thus, the range of levels may be restricted by technical capabilities or pragmatism. For instance, in a study assessing user preferences in the provision of *in vitro* fertilisation services one of the attributes was chance of taking home a baby. This attribute ranged in levels from 5% to 35%.[18] To assign a level of success in the questionnaire much higher than 35% would have been unrealistic and possibly unethical.

Stage 3: Which scenarios to present?

Scenarios are then drawn up describing all possible service (or outcome) configurations given the characteristics and levels chosen. The number of scenarios increases with the number of characteristics and levels. Rarely can all the scenarios generated be included in the questionnaire, and experimental designs, using computer software (such as SPSS *ORTHOPLAN* and *SPEED*) or catalogues, are used to reduce the scenarios to a manageable level while still being able to estimate benefits for all possible scenarios.[26,27] The reduced combination of scenarios are orthogonal in design. This ensures a lack of correlation between attribute levels, and thus ensures that the effect of individual attributes can be isolated in the analysis.

Stage 4: Establishing preferences

Preferences for scenarios included in the questionnaire are elicited using one of three methods: discrete choices; rating; or ranking. Using the discrete choice approach, respondents are presented with a number of choices which vary with respect to the levels of a number of predefined characteristics. For each choice respondents are asked to choose their preferred one. They may be asked in a direct choice question such as do you prefer A or B, or graded such as 'definitely prefer A', 'probably prefer A', 'no preference', 'probably prefer B', 'definitely prefer B'.[8] The rating method requires the respondents to assign a score, of say 1 to 10, to each of the scenarios defined from the experimental design. This is shown in the example described below.[20] Within ranking exercises respondents are presented with the scenarios presented from the experimental design and asked to list them in order of preference from most (least) preferred to least (most) preferred. The report by Ryan *et al*.[8] provides a review of the application of discrete choices, rating and ranking conjoint analysis exercises in healthcare.

Stage 5: Data analysis

Regression techniques are used to analyse responses, and a benefit (also known as satisfaction or utility) function is estimated. The method of data collection (rating, ranking or discrete choices) will determine the appropriate regression method.[28] The benefit function to be estimated can be specified as:

$$B = \beta_0 + \beta_1 X_1 + \beta_2 X_2 + \beta_3 X_3 + \cdots + \beta_n X_n \tag{1}$$

where B is the benefit from the given healthcare service or intervention being considered, X_j ($j = 1, 2 \ldots, n$) are the levels of the attributes, β_0 is the constant term and β_j ($j = 1, 2 \ldots, n$) are the coefficients (weights) of the model to be estimated. It should be noted that while conjoint analysis has traditionally been used to measure utility from process attributes and non-health outcomes, the above utility function can also be used to generate quality weights within the QALY paradigm. For an example of this *see* Netten *et al.*[29]

From this estimated equation it is possible to estimate:

- *impact of individual characteristics* – the importance of a marginal change in the different characteristics of the service, as indicated by both the significance of the coefficients, and their relative size. This allows the policy maker to observe the impact of each individual characteristic on overall benefit
- *how people are willing to trade between characteristics* – this is shown by the ratio of any two coefficients. For example, β_3/β_2 indicates how much of β_2 an individual is willing to give up to have more of β_3. If a price proxy is included as an attribute, then it is possible to estimate how much money an individual is willing to give up for a marginal improvement in the level of any given attribute (i.e. willingness to pay – WTP). For example, in the study concerned with the preferences of South Australians for hospital services, Medicare levy was included as an attribute,[25] in the study concerned with the importance Isle of Wight residents place on reducing waiting time for elective surgery, travel costs were included as an attribute[21] and in the study looking at the value of *in vitro* fertilisation (IVF), the cost of an IVF attempt was included as an attribute.[18] Conjoint analysis represents an alternative approach to eliciting WTP measures compared with the more direct WTP approaches that have been used in the literature to estimate monetary measures of benefit
- *total benefit scores for alternative ways of providing healthcare* – this is estimated by multiplying the coefficient (or weight) for any given attribute by the level of that attribute. The scores enable health service scenarios to be ranked against one another, which is particularly useful in a priority setting context.

An application in general practice

In what follows, an application is presented from the area of primary care. For more information on this study *see* Ryan *et al.*[20] The structure from the previous section is followed to guide the reader through the stages of a conjoint analysis study. The aim of the study was to elicit the value of introducing a patient health card (PHC) within a general practice setting.

Background

A randomised controlled trial was carried out at a health centre in a small town in Scotland, to test whether the availability of comprehensive and up-to-date information (in the form of increased access to information) on patient held electronic records would bring benefits to patients and enable health professionals to provide a more efficient service. Half of all patients at the health centre were issued credit card sized optical cards holding their complete medical records. The remainder continued without a PHC. At each healthcare location where it was used, the card interfaced to the local computer system. This enabled health professionals to exchange information via the medium of the card. The patient could view the information on the card at any time using a stand-alone patient access system, one of which was located in the waiting area at the health centre. The type of information that was readily available on the PHC included medical details of the patient, information on drugs prescribed and previous medical history. In addition, the card could be used to access general medical information, for example on stopping smoking or information about certain conditions. One hundred individuals from Inverurie Health Centre were asked to take part in the conjoint analysis study.

Stages 1 and 2

The policy question identified the characteristics to be included in the conjoint analysis study – the value of introducing a PHC. The PHC was evaluated with respect to three other aspects of general practice: number of days between making a non-urgent appointment and seeing a doctor; waiting time in reception between time of appointment and seeing a doctor; and whether the patient is usually seen by a doctor of their choice. These attributes were established by reviewing the literature on patient preferences for attributes of general practice, using the results of a survey looking at patient satisfaction with the Inverurie Health Centre and by talking to general practitioners. The attributes and their levels are shown in Table 21.2.

Table 21.2:   Attributes and levels in the conjoint analysis study

Attributes		Levels
• Waiting time between making a non-urgent appointment and seeing a doctor	Days	1 day, 3 days
• How long a patient would usually expect to wait in reception between the time of the appointment and seeing a doctor	Wait	5 minutes, 15 minutes, 25 minutes
• Whether the patient is usually seen by the doctor of choice or by any one of the doctors in the practice	Doctor	0 = any one of the doctors 1 = doctor of choice
• Whether the practice gives the patient a health card or not	Health card	0 = no health card offered, 1 = health card offered

Stage 3

The attributes and levels in Table 21.2 gave rise to 24 possible scenarios (or general practice configurations) ($3^1 \times 2^3$). A component of the statistical package SPSS (Orthoplan) was used to reduce the possible number of scenarios to a manageable level while still allowing preferences to be inferred for all combinations of levels and attributes. Using this design the 24 possible scenarios were reduced to eight (Table 21.3).

Stage 4

Each respondent was presented with these eight scenarios and asked, for each, to state their level of preference on a scale of one to eight where one indicated 'dislike very much' and eight indicated 'like very much'. Checks for internal

Table 21.3:   General practice descriptions used in the conjoint analysis study

Description	Time to appointment (days)	Waiting time (minutes)	Which doctor you see	Patient health card
Practice 1	1	5	May be any doctor	No
Practice 2	3	25	May be any doctor	Yes
Practice 3	3	15	Doctor of your choice	No
Practice 4	1	25	Doctor of your choice	No
Practice 5	3	5	Doctor of your choice	Yes
Practice 6	3	5	May be any doctor	No
Practice 7	1	5	Doctor of your choice	Yes
Practice 8	1	15	May be any doctor	Yes

consistency were included. It was assumed that, all other things being equal, respondents prefer shorter waiting times in reception and fewer days' wait before their appointment. No *a priori* assumptions were made about preferences for a PHC or whether patients prefer to see a doctor of their choice. Given these assumptions, practices 1, 7 and 8 should have been preferred to practices 6, 5 and 2 respectively, and therefore given a higher rating.

Stage 5

The following benefit equation was estimated for consistent respondents:

$$B = \beta_0 + \beta_1 \text{Days} + \beta_2 \text{Wait} + \beta_3 \text{Doctor} + \beta_4 \text{Healthcard} \qquad (1)$$

where B is the benefit score or preference score for a general practice with a given level of each attribute and the explanatory variables are as defined in Table 21.2. Coefficients β_1 to β_4 may be interpreted as weights for the different attributes, thus indicating the relative importance of the different attributes. When interpreting these weights it is important to be aware of the unit of measurement: β_1 is in days, β_2 minutes, and β_3 and β_4 represent a unit change from having no choice to having choice or having no patient health card to having a card. Benefit scores were estimated for different general practice configurations shown in Table 21.3.

Results

Sixty-seven respondents returned the questionnaire, of whom 51 completed the conjoint analysis section. High levels of consistency were found, with test 1 (comparing practice 1 and 6) and test 2 (comparing practices 7 and 5) having 80% consistency rates, and test 3 (comparing practice 8 and 2) a 96% consistency rate. The higher level of consistency for test 3 may be explained by the fact that in this test both 'Days' and 'Wait' varied, compared with the other tests where only 'Days' varied.

Impact of individual characteristics

Table 21.4 presents the regression results. The positive and significant signs of choice and PHC shows that respondents preferred having these attributes than not. Moving from not having a doctor of your choice to having a doctor of your choice will increase benefits by 0.816 and having a PHC will increase benefits by 0.063. The negative and significant signs on 'Days' and 'Wait' indicate that the higher the levels of these two attributes, the lower the benefits. The negative coefficient of 0.291 on 'Days' indicates a unit increase in days (for instance from 1 day to 2 days) will reduce the benefit score by 0.291.

Table 21.4:   Results from the regression analysis

Attributes	Coefficient (weight)	p-value
Constant	3.30	0.001
Time (days)	−0.291	0.001
Wait (minutes)	−0.220	0.001
Doctor of choice (0 = no, 1 = yes)	0.172	0.001
Health card (0 = no, 1 = yes)	0.063	0.006

How people are willing to trade between characteristics

Individuals are prepared to wait more than an extra half a day to see the doctor of their choice. This has been calculated from the ratio of the coefficients of 'Doctor' and 'Days' (0.172/0.291 = 0.59, i.e. approximately half a day). We can use this same measure of willingness to wait to see how the respondents value the PHC. From the ratio of 'Healthcard' to 'Days' (0.063/0.291) we can see that the value placed on the PHC (0.2 of a day) is less than that placed on seeing the doctor of their choice.

Total benefit scores for alternative ways of providing healthcare

Total benefit scores for different combinations of attributes can be calculated by inserting different combinations of levels of attributes into the regression model from equation (1) (Table 21.5). These total scores for each combination of attributes can then be ranked in order of preference, with a higher score indicating a higher preference. The most favoured general practice (i.e. that ranked first)

Table 21.5:   Satisfaction (utility) scores for the eight general practices presented in the conjoint analysis questionnaire

Description	Days	Wait	Doctor	Healthcard	Benefit (satisfaction or utility) score*	Ranking
Practice 1	1	5	No (0)	Yes (1)	1.769	2nd
Practice 2	3	25	No (0)	Yes (1)	−3.15	8th
Practice 3	3	15	Yes (1)	No (0)	−0.84	16th
Practice 4	1	25	Yes (1)	No (0)	−2.459	7th
Practice 5	3	5	Yes (1)	Yes (1)	1.422	3rd
Practice 6	3	5	No (0)	No (0)	1.187	4th
Practice 7	1	5	Yes (1)	Yes (1)	2.004	1st
Practice 8	1	15	No (0)	Yes (1)	−0.368	5th

*Benefit score = 3.30 − 0.291Days − 0.220Wait + 0.172 Doctor + 0.063 Healthcard.

would be a practice which had only a 1-day wait for an appointment, a 5-minute wait in reception, doctor of choice and offered a PHC. The least preferred practice, Practice 2, has a healthcard, but is poor with regard to all the other attributes which have been shown to be more important than having a healthcard.

Conclusion

This chapter proposes conjoint analysis as a rigorous survey technique for eliciting the views of patients and people in the community on healthcare. The application presented here shows the potential uses of the technique. With particular reference to the application, while the patients did value the PHC scheme (the coefficient was positive and statistically significant), the strength of that value was low compared with other aspects of the primary care service. The nature of the conjoint questionnaire with its inherent trade-offs produced a data set which enables us to draw these types of conclusions in a way that simple patient satisfaction data would not have.

At a more general level, conjoint analysis is a rigorous survey technique for eliciting patient/community views in healthcare. The technique has been successfully applied in healthcare, and shows great potential as an instrument for establishing patient and community preferences (as well as those of clinicians and policy makers). Important areas of future research relate to experimental design, alternative methods of data collection and analysis and investigation of the underlying axioms of economic theory. Collaborative work with psychologists and qualitative researchers will prove useful when investigating these issues.[30]

References

1 Secretaries of State for Health, Wales, Northern Ireland and Scotland (1989) *Working for Patients*. HMSO, London.
2 NHS (1992) *Local Voices: the views of local people in purchasing for health*. NHSME, London.
3 Secretaries of State for Health, Wales, Northern Ireland and Scotland (1989) *Promoting Better Health*. HMSO, London.
4 Secretary of State for Health (1989) *The Health of the Nation*. HMSO, London.
5 Scottish Office Department of Health (1992) *The Patient's Charter: what users think*. HMSO, Edinburgh.

6 NHS Management Executive (1992) *Local Voices: the views of local people in purchasing for health*. NHSME, London.

7 Cleary P (1999) The increasing importance of patient surveys. *BMJ*. **319**: 720–1.

8 Ryan M, Scott DA, Reeves C *et al.* (2001) Eliciting public preferences for health care: a systematic review of techniques. *Health Technol Assess*. **5(5)**. (www.ncchta.org)

9 Luce D and Tukey J (1964) Simultaneous conjoint measurement: a new type of fundamental measurement. *J Mathematical Psychology*. **1**: 1–27.

10 Anderson N (1977) Functional measurement and psycho-physical judgement. *Psycholog Rev*. **77**: 153–70.

11 Cattin P and Wittink D (1982) Commercial use of conjoint analysis: a survey. *J Marketing*. **46**: 44–53.

12 (1988) *J Transport Economics Policy*. **22**.

13 Adamowicz W, Louviere J and Williams M (1994) Combining revealed preference and stated preference methods for valuing environmental amenities. *J Environmental Economics Management*. **6**: 271–92.

14 Bryan S, Buxton M, Sheldon R and Grant A (1998) Magnetic resonance imaging for the investigation of knee injuries: an investigation of preference. *Health Economics*. **7**: 595–604.

15 Propper C (1991) Contingent valuation of time spent on NHS waiting list. *The Economic Journal*. **100**: 193–9.

16 Propper C (1995) The disutility of time spent on the United Kingdom's National Health Service waiting lists. *J Hum Resources*. **30**: 677–700.

17 Ratcliffe J and Buxton M (1999) Patients' preferences regarding the process and outcomes of life saving technology: an application of conjoint analysis to liver transplantation. *International J Technol Assess Health Care*. **15**: 340–51.

18 Ryan M (1999) Using conjoint analysis to go beyond health outcomes: an application to in vitro fertilisation. *Soc Sci Med*. **8**: 535–46.

19 Van der Pol M and Cairns J (1998) Establishing preferences for blood transfusion support: an application of conjoint analysis. *J Health Services Research Management*. **3**: 70–6.

20 Ryan M, McIntosh E and Shackley P (1998) Using conjoint analysis to assess consumer preferences in primary care: an application to the patient health card. *Health Expectations*. **1**: 117–29.

21 Ryan M, McIntosh E, Dean T and Old P (2000) Trade-offs between location and waiting times in the provision of health care: the case of elective surgery on the Isle of Wight. *J Public Health Med*. **22**: 202–10.

22 Farrar S, Ryan M, Ross D and Ludbrook A (2000) Using discrete choice modelling in priority setting: an application to clinical service developments. *Soc Sci Med*. **50**: 63–75.

23 Ryan M and Hughes J (1997) Using conjoint analysis to value surgical versus medical management of miscarriage. *Health Economics*. **6**: 261–73.

24 Ryan M and Farrar S (2000) Eliciting preferences for health care using conjoint analysis. *BMJ*. **320**: 1530–3.

25 Jan S, Mooney G, Ryan M, Bruggemann K and Alexander K (2000) What type of hospital services do we want to use? The preferences of the South Australian public. *Australian and New Zealand J Public Health*. **24**: 64–70.

26 Kocur G, Alder T, Hyman W and Aunet B (1982) *Guide to Forecasting Travel Demand with Direct Utility Assessment*. US Department of Transportation, Washington DC.

27 Bradley M (1991) *User's Manual for the SPEED Version 2.1: stated preference experiment*. Hague Consulting Group, Hague.

28 Greene W (1993) *Econometric Analysis*. Prentice Hall, Englewood Cliffs, NJ.
29 Netten A, Ryan M, Smith P *et al.* (2002) *The Development of a Measure of Social Care Outcome for Older People*. Discussion Paper 1690/2. Personal Social Services Research Unit, Canterbury.
30 Ryan M, Bate A, Eastmond C and Ludbrook A (2001) Using discrete choice experiments to elicit preferences. *Qual Health Care*. **10:** 155–60.

CHAPTER 22

Making the trade-off between efficiency and equity

Charles Normand

In many cases, it is possible that the largest health gain may not result from services directed to those who are less well off or in poorer health. A trade-off is often necessary between efficiency (in the sense of maximising some index of health) and a more equal or fairer distribution of services. This trade-off is not easy. It is necessary to have a clear and agreed concept of equity, the ability to measure equity and an agreed basis for the extent to which equity factors will be weighted in the choice process. It is also important to be clear whether the inequity in any system is the result of a failure to pursue efficiency properly, or whether equity and efficiency must be traded off. This chapter explores the difficulties in this area.

Key points

- Equity and efficiency are not always conflicting objectives – as illness is concentrated in poorer parts of the population, so also is the capacity to benefit.
- Many observed inequalities in health are outside of the influence of personal health services.
- Equity and fairness are a difficult concept, and we need to be clear what we mean before we can take action to improve the distribution of services.
- Some approaches to equity are highly controversial, such as giving low priority to those who have already had a 'fair innings'.
- Equity can be explicitly included in economic evaluation or an assessment of equity effects can be carried out in parallel.
- There can be no exercise trading off equity and efficiency that does not worsen the overall measured health of the population.

Chapter sections
- **Introduction**
- **What do we mean by equity and fairness**
- **Equity in what?**
- **Giving people the same chance in life – the idea of the fair innings**
- **Trading off equity and efficiency**
- **Taking account of equity in planning and developing health services**
- **Pursuing equity in the application of economic evaluation**
- **Conclusion**

Introduction

Economic analysis in health and healthcare is undertaken to help governments and other heath agencies to achieve better their health policy goals. Where explicit goals are specified, it is common for two to dominate – improving the health status of the population and fairness or equity. Most health economists share these objectives, and work to maximise the impact of services on health and equity. Economists argue that choices must be made – it is not possible to achieve everything you want. To some extent it is possible to use resources in ways that are both efficient and equitable. However, beyond a certain point more equity is likely to be achieved only with less improvement in health. In other words, we can choose to trade-off efficiency (the achievement of better health) and equity (the fairer distribution of health).

It is useful to distinguish between the structure and intended operation of a health system and the way it actually works.[1] Health systems that provide universal access to (important components of) healthcare might be expected to give priority to poorer, sicker people, and should reduce health inequalities. It is well known that health systems fail to meet the objective of access according to need, but in some senses the failure to be efficient and equitable requires action not to change the structure, but to make the system work as intended. It will be argued that this sometimes means maximising efficiency in the sense of ensuring that services go to those likely to benefit most. Only sometimes will it mean pursuing equity at the expense of efficiency.

Systems with high levels of user fees and payments, or which rely on private insurance, allocate services to those who can mobilise the necessary resources, who are likely to be in need of services, but not necessarily those most in need.[2] It is difficult to identify a clear role for economic evaluation in this case, as there is no decision maker. Economic evaluation is only useful when there is some process that replaces the allocation of resources that would result from the normal (if imperfect) operation of a market.

What do we mean by equity and fairness

Equity and fairness are complex concepts. A large literature exists just on what is meant by the terms.[3,4] The concepts carry strong moral overtones. Few people argue openly in favour of widening gaps in health between the rich and poor. The very terminology makes it difficult to be opposed to fairness.

People are often unclear as to what they mean by equity or fairness, and it is important to define the concepts and desired outcomes more precisely and give careful thought to how they should be measured.[5,6] There can be many reasons why health and access to healthcare are unequal. Some people happen to be born with diseases or disabilities, or the predisposition to become ill. Some people are just unlucky, and become ill. Those without jobs (or in dangerous jobs) or those without proper housing may live in risky or unhealthy conditions. Others take risks, such as smoking or rock climbing which can lead to bad outcomes. And some people would benefit from treatment or care, but cannot find the resources to pay for it.

The two classic concepts of equity are treating equals the same (horizontal equity) and treating unequals differently (vertical equity). Apart from problems of measurement, the first appears to be relatively simple. However, it does beg the question, in what respects are people equals? Take a simple example. If two people have the same degree of loss of sight from cataract, and would have the same improvement in sight from surgery, but one has 10 years of expected life and the other 2 years, are they in equal need? Economists normally say no, as the capacity to benefit is affected by the duration of effect. Concerns are often raised that taking into account duration of benefit discriminates against older people, as in general younger people have longer to enjoy the benefits of treatment. However, most people agree that some allowance must be made for duration of effect − if we take the *reductio ad absurdum* case of a benefit of days against that of years, few would argue against priority for the longer duration. It is perhaps odd that many non-economists argue that we should take account only of very large differences in duration of effect. Perhaps this is best thought about as the degree to which we take account of the unequal needs of unequals.

Vertical equity requires that differences in needs be taken into account in setting priorities. There are obvious problems in defining the differences, but also the extent to which different needs justify different responses. An important issue is how need should be defined. In common usage we tend to consider need as the size of a problem. However, someone with a serious problem that will in no way respond to treatment, has a problem, but no need for treatment services. Should the size of a problem be taken into account in setting priorities? Many would argue that it is only fair to help those with the largest problems, but economists tend to focus on the size of the solution and not the size of the problem. This can lead to very different perspectives on horizontal equity, with economists interested in identifying large health gains and others large health problems.

To some extent it is necessary to draw on the population consensus about what decisions are fair. An important approach uses the concept of the veil of ignorance – what decision would you make if you knew all the facts, but did not know who you are?[7] In effect something is fair if it would be chosen by someone self-interested but ignorant about who they are.

Equity in what?

It is self-evident that we cannot successfully equalise health. Many factors are beyond the control of either health promotion or treatment. Even though we cannot equalise the levels of health, we can aim to ensure that services are available on an equitable basis, whatever we mean by this. Should we always give priority to interventions that narrow differences in health over those that widen them? Would we even do this when the potential gains to the worst off would be minute, and those to others life changing? Is inequality between groups in society (for example, the better health of white people or the better health of women) a more serious problem than variation that is less systematic? Is poor health more of a problem for poorer people (whose welfare is worse in many other ways) than for richer ones? These are arguments for aiming at equity of wider concepts of welfare and not simply on health, but health services aim mainly to make differences in the narrower dimension of health.[8]

Although we cannot make health equal, an objective may nevertheless be to make access to services more equitable. This could be based either on the degree to which people have health problems, or the degree to which they are likely to benefit from care. Should account be taken of refusal to comply with advice on health? Should we give priority to those in need even when their illness is clearly the result of health damaging behaviour, such as smoking or skiing? Should the aim be to equalise the levels of health or the opportunity to enjoy good health? Is there a difference between those whose health damaging behaviour is the result of ignorance and that due to plain stupidity?

The argument about people's behaviour has two dimensions. First, is there an equally strong moral argument for priority if the problem were clearly self-imposed and avoidable? Second, as those who smoke are less likely to enjoy health gains following treatment, should quitting be a requirement before treatment is offered? The second is really an efficiency argument – we should not give priority to treatment that, however much the person is ill, is not likely to make them better.

Giving people the same chance in life – the idea of the fair innings

A recent debate has emerged on the idea of a 'fair innings'. The idea is based on a sporting analogy. In a game of cricket a batsman who is out after scoring 100 leaves the field to praise from all. It is no tragedy to be out in these circumstances. A player who is out without scoring a single run may be considered to have had a tragic experience. This is interpreted by Williams[8,9] in terms of a right to a quota of quality adjusted life years. Harris[10] has given some support to the idea by contrasting the misfortune of death in old age and the tragedy of a young death. The principle is that those who have already done their fair share of living would get lower priority in resources to extend further their lives, or to enhance their quality. Some attempts have been made to quantify this based on the declared preferences of people who respond to surveys.[11]

The idea of the fair innings is strongly opposed by campaigners for better services for older people.[12] There is also some reason to be sceptical about the evidence from population surveys, as it is very difficult to frame questions in this area. However, the issue remains, is it fair for access to future services to be independent of someone's previous luck or enjoyment? On the other hand, is it really feasible to use previous quality adjusted life lived as a basis for rationing. There would certainly be strong incentives to emphasise the unhappiness of your childhood, your poor health in previous years and your need to be given priority in the future.

Trading off equity and efficiency

Economists often focus on the trade-off between efficiency and equity. The need to do this occurs only when, for whatever reason, it is cheaper to improve health in those who already enjoy better health or those who are relatively well off. This is important, as most people (and most decision makers) would choose more equity in preference to less so long as there is no other sacrifice. The equity efficiency choice exists only when to gain greater fairness or equity we have to agree to a lower level of health overall.

Take an example based on experience in an urban area in England. Due to differences in referral rates, people in the poorest part of the district had the highest rates of treatable coronary heart disease, but were getting less treatment than those from more prosperous parts. In effect, those with the least capacity to benefit were getting more, and those likely to benefit more received less. A closer examination made it clear why this was occurring. The barrier to access to treatment was access to assessment, in particular to angiography. There was no social class difference in treatment rates for those who had had the relevant tests and who had been found suitable for treatment. However, there was a large difference in access to assessment and diagnosis. Despite disease being more serious in elderly people, younger ones were much more likely to be offered tests.

In this case, the allocation of resources is inefficient (as more improvement in health could be achieved within the existing budget by reallocation). Greater efficiency would also lead to greater equity. Being ill or at risk is a necessary condition for being able to benefit from treatment, so that it is often the case that those who can benefit most are those with low incomes and above average morbidity. On the face of it, this means that it is likely, in a system that is designed to provide services based on capacity to benefit, that inefficiencies will also lead to inequity. It is the failure to deliver and not a failure of intention that leads to the problem.

In some cases it is more expensive to treat poorer people, as they may need longer in hospital. There are also cases where there are higher costs of running a prevention programme for poorer people. For example, those attending for screening programmes tend to be those who are richer and have less disease. Recruiting those from poorer families may be important, as there are likely to be more diseases detected, but it may cost more to organise such a programme.

Take another example of urban and rural populations, who have different perinatal mortality rates. It is common for rural areas to have worse rates of such deaths, so we might expect the efforts of public health and health services to focus on reducing this difference. However, it is also likely that the cost of lowering the rate of perinatal deaths in rural areas will be higher, mainly because providers cannot deliver healthcare at such efficient levels, and professionals spend time travelling. This means that a given expenditure might do more to lower the number of deaths if applied in the urban area. There are several reasons for this, not least that it is usually more expensive to provide personal health services to dispersed and sparse populations.

A real choice might be to lower the number of deaths by 100 if the focus is on urban areas but only by 80 if the same funds were spent on the rural programme. A difficult choice faces policy makers – spend the money on the urban areas and more deaths are prevented, but at the same time the disparity between urban and rural areas would become wider. Are we really concerned about the relative numbers of deaths, or only the absolute number of avoidable deaths? If we are worried about the relative number, why is this?

Of course we would all like to see both fewer deaths and less inequality, but in this example, for any given spending we cannot avoid making the difficult choice between a more efficient intervention (i.e. fewer deaths) and a more equitable one. Is the additional fairness worth 20 deaths? This is the serious version of pursuing an objective of equity and fairness. Much of the public debate concerns only cases where there is really no dilemma – where there is really no trade-off, and current inequities arise through a lack of effort.

The above example is not just made up to illustrate the case – it is based on a real choice that was faced by a health agency in the 1980s. The geographical area concerned had one town with about half the population, and a very large rural population, mainly engaged in farming of quite marginal land. To provide services of equal effectiveness requires much more resource in this difficult to serve population.

These examples aim to shed light on two aspects of equity. In the first, it is really a question of being more effective in doing what we intend to do. The objectives of efficiency and equity are not clashing, and the inefficiency brings with it an unintended inequity. It is not obvious in this example that the cause of greater equity is well served by focusing on this – as the failure is to do what is intended, the problem of inequity may be seen as a management failure. As suggested above, if the cause of inequity is not failure of policy but rather of implementation it is not clear whether the best solutions lie in focusing on the resulting inequalities or injustice.

Taking account of equity in planning and developing health services

It can be useful to distinguish within the health sector between structures that lead to unequal access to services and the failure of health systems to work as they are planned to. Countries with tax or social insurance funding for healthcare normally aim to provide nearly equal access to important services. The rules normally state that care should be offered on the basis of need and not on income or ability to pay. The reality is often different, as there may be user charges (whether official or unofficial), medicines may not be available at the hospitals, staff may be rude and careless with poorer patients, and buildings may be in a poor state of repair. The design may be for a system of equal access, but the reality is that those with more money get better access. However, the answer to inequity is, again, to plan and manage the service in line with its stated aims.

This may be contrasted to systems that do not aim to provide equal access. In the USA access depends on income, employment, age and disease. Those who are employed and insured get excellent services. Those who are very poor or old get free or subsidised services, many of which are very good. Those with renal failure get free dialysis. However, those with low paid jobs, and no insurance may be excluded from many parts of the system. Even if each part of the system were to work as planned, the system does not aim to provide the same health-care opportunities to all users. The answer to any undesired inequity in this case requires changes in the system objectives and structures, or changes in the overall distribution of income and wealth.

This is not necessarily to argue the superiority of systems that aim to be equitable but fail, over ones without such an aim. In the end it is the outcome and not the intention that affects patients. What is important is that the logic of how to intervene is different, depending on objectives and the extent to which inequity is a symptom of failure to pursue objectives effectively.

Pursuing equity in the application of economic evaluation

It should be clear from the argument above that the trade-off between efficiency and equity is an issue only in some cases. In many cases greater economic efficiency will in itself increase equity, and no adjustment to take account of equity issues is needed. Taking equity into account specifically can have a role only where there is a trade-off between more health gain and a fairer distribution of the gain.

There are several possible mechanisms to include equity concerns into the evaluation of services and the setting of priorities – the simplest is to carry out economic evaluation in the normal way, but to check for any undesirable or undesired effects on distribution. *Ad hoc* measures can be taken to change decisions if difficulties are found. The alternative is to apply equity weights to the measures of outputs, so as to include equity directly in the evaluation process. Equity weighted quality adjusted life years (QALYs) have been proposed[13-16] and the same approach can be taken to other benefit measures. The advantages of this approach are in the consistency and formal consideration of the equity issues, but it is necessary to derive and apply explicit weights.

There is a long history of trying to build equity considerations into economic evaluation, probably starting in the 1960s. Weisbrod[17] suggested that we examine past decisions and infer weights from the difference between what maximises efficiency and the decisions actually taken. This has several worrying risks – not least that past errors are used to inform future decisions. It is also a bit optimistic to think that past decisions were taken on a rational basis that at least implicitly took proper account of the relevant efficiency and equity issues.

More recent attempts to weight outcomes for equity rely on data from surveys and population opinion. As with the case of surveys of opinion for fair innings weights, such data should be treated with great caution. The real problem is how to ask questions that are properly understood by respondents. Returning to the example of perinatal mortality, we can imagine two ways of asking the question.

- Are you in favour of giving priority to reducing inequalities in child deaths between urban and rural areas as well as reducing deaths overall?
- Are you in favour of letting an extra 20 babies die in order to reduce the difference between death rates in rural and urban areas in this district?

At a guess more people would answer yes to the first than would to the second. Similar problems arise in framing fair innings questions. There is, therefore, a risk that problems in framing the questions play at least some part in determining the patterns of answers and therefore the equity weights. Chapter 28 considers these issues in more detail.

Advocates of equity weighting would argue, quite rightly, that the objective is not to find the perfect answers, but rather to do better than we do at present. It may be a case where the best is the enemy of the good. If there is a real desire for equity issues to take priority, and the choices are really there, then doing it badly may dominate not doing it at all.

Conclusion

There is not always a real trade-off between efficiency and equity. Where capacity to benefit from services is concentrated in those with the worst health, then the appropriate action is likely to be to make the system work as planned. Trading off efficiency for greater equity is an issue only when, for some reason, the greatest health gain is available for those who are healthier or wealthier.

Defining equity is difficult and controversial. Without a clearer definition it is difficult to evaluate the extent of the problem, and the appropriate responses to it. Particular controversy arises when equity is defined in terms of giving everyone a chance to have a 'fair innings'. Even when the problem can be defined clearly, there are problems in deciding what weight to give to equity considerations. Some guide can be derived from population surveys and studies, but there remain difficulties in such research. In particular it is difficult to frame questions that are understood by respondents in the way intended.

Despite these difficulties, it is clear that there is a widespread desire to reduce health inequalities, and to ensure that the system is not simply efficient, but also fair. We can use existing tools to take equity goals into account in economic evaluation, and it may be better to start using such approaches rather than waiting for the perfect system.

References

1   Aday LA, Begley CE, Lairson DR and Slater CH (1998) *Evaluating the Healthcare System: effectiveness, efficiency and equity*. Health Administration Press, Chicago.

2   Akin J (1986) *Fees for Service and Concern for Equity for the Poor*. Technical Note Series. World Bank, Washington DC.

3   Musgrave P (1986) Measurement of equity in health. *World Health Statistics Quarterly*. **39**.

4   Mooney G (1987) What does equity in healthcare mean? *World Health Statistics Quarterly*. **40**.

5   O'Donnell O and Propper C (1991) Equity and the distribution of UK National Health Service resources. *J Health Economics*. **10**: 1–19.

6   van Doorslaer E, Wagstaff A and Rutten F (1993) *Equity in the Finance and Delivery of Healthcare: an international perspective*. Oxford University Press, Oxford.

7   Rawls J (1971) *A Theory of Justice*. Harvard University Press, Cambridge, MA.

8   Williams A (1997) Intergenerational equity and exploration of the 'fair innings' argument. *Health Economics*. **6**: 117–32.

9   Williams A (1998) If we are going to get a fair innings someone will need to keep the score! In: ML Barer, TE Getzen and GL Stoddart (eds) *Health, Health Care and Health Economics: perspectives on distribution*. John Wiley and Sons, Chichester.

10 Harris J (1985) *The Value of Life*. Routledge and Kegan Paul, London.

11 Tsuchiya A (1999) Age-related preferences and age weighting health benefits. *Soc Sci Med*. **48(2)**: 267–76.

12 Evans JG (2000) Marjory Warren Lecture: service and research for an ageing population. *Age Ageing*. **29**: 5–8.

13 Gafni A and Birch S (1991) Equity considerations in utility based measures of health outcomes in economic appraisals: an adjustment algorithm. *J Health Economics*. **10**: 329–42.

14 Wagstaff A (1991) QALYs and the equity–efficiency trade-off. *J Health Economics*. **10**: 21–41.

15 Bleichrodt H (1997) Health utility indices and equity considerations. *J Health Economics*. **16(1)**: 65–91.

16 Nord E, Pinto JL, Richardson J, Menzel P and Ubel P (1999) Incorporating societal concerns for fairness in numerical valuation of health programmes. *Health Economics*. **8**: 25–39.

17 Weisbrod BA (1968) Income distribution effects and benefit cost analysis. In: SB Chase (ed) *Problems in Public Expenditure Analysis*. Brookings Institute, Washington DC, 177–209.

CHAPTER 23

Patients' rights, NHS rationing and the law

Christopher Newdick

The legal dimension of rationing is often overlooked. This chapter explores the evolution of the influence of the courts in this area and its relationship with the economic input into the decision-making process.

Key points
- The position of the courts has changed from a passive observer, submissive to the directives of managers and clinicians, to a more active role.
- The impact of the courts has been to require resource decisions to be made within a more explicit framework without necessarily directing how that framework should be constructed.
- The law directs that rationing policies must enable patients to have access to a review of their case if their need is exceptional. Blanket bans are not acceptable.
- Due to the GP's Terms of Service, the legal perspectives on rationing in secondary and primary care are very different.
- By themselves, efficiency concerns do not fit well within the legal framework particularly with the GP's Terms of Service obligation to treat on the basis of need.

Chapter sections
- **Introduction**
- **Is rationing lawful?**
- **Rationing at health authority level**
- **Rationing at the national level: 'guidance', 'directions' and the status of NICE**
- **Rationing in primary care**
- **Conclusion**

Introduction

How does the law affect NHS rationing and does it allow health economics to resolve the allocation of limited resources? The first case to address this issue was brought in 1980, and for the rest of the decade the courts remained entirely passive and deferential to decisions by clinicians and managers. The 1990s were marked by two developments. First, following the purchaser/provider split, the focus of rationing decisions in secondary care moved from clinicians to health authorities. Second, a much more inquisitive approach was adopted by the courts which was to impose new duties on health authorities. As we shall see, general practice remained largely untouched.

This chapter reviews the development of rationing within a legal framework from the health authority, national and primary care perspectives. It demonstrates how the law has required resource decisions to be made within a more explicit framework without necessarily directing how that framework should be constructed.

Is rationing lawful?

The National Health Service Act 1977 is the foundation of the NHS and most relevant to the rationing question (although other statutes also govern the service). Sections 1 and 3 impose a duty on the Secretary of State to promote 'a comprehensive health service' and to provide certain specified services such as 'hospital accommodation, medical, dental and ambulance services' and so on. Claims to resources made under the Act are often made in the law of judicial review. Judicial review considers whether a public authority has complied with the duties imposed upon it by parliament. From the rationing perspective, the patient claims that the relevant authority has failed to fulfil the duty imposed upon it and the court should require the authority to take the decision all over again. (Notice that the court cannot take the decision on behalf of the authority.) A number of patients have challenged decisions to deny them access to care. They help to explain the evolution of the law on rationing. We discuss two cases that demonstrate a very passive judicial approach to NHS rationing, followed by two that reflect a more interventionist judicial attitude.

Judicial non-interference

The Hincks case

The first claim to NHS resources arose in the case of Hincks in 1980 over access to orthopaedic care. The Secretary of State acknowledged the need for better facilities in Birmingham and said additional resources would be made available. However, he was unable to provide the funding promised and action was brought by patients who would have benefited from the facilities. Lord Denning said that the 1977 Act imposes no specific duty on the Secretary of State. His duty is to 'promote', but not to 'provide' a comprehensive service. Further, the duty is not absolute, it is always subject to the resources made available by the Treasury and to current government economic policy. Obviously, this creates a very insubstantial basis on which patients can claim rights to NHS resources.

The Collier case

Hincks was followed in 1988 by the Collier case, perhaps the most distressing abdication of judicial responsibility one is likely to find. Here, a boy aged 4 years had a hole in the heart and was top of his consultant's list. He was likely to die without treatment. Yet, for reasons that were never clearly explained to the Court, his operation was cancelled time and again so that his life was in danger. Application was made for judicial review. Astonishingly, basing itself on Hincks, the court said it had no role to play in this case. Understandably, courts have no special expertise in these matters. Here, however, the court refused even to ask why the boy was being effectively abandoned by the responsible authority. For example, was the reason for the situation that other more urgent patients needed treatment first (unlikely!), or that it was impossible to transfer him elsewhere? The court meekly accepted that resources constraints can have unfortunate consequences for patients. Had things stopped here, it would have been almost impossible to argue that law could ever regulate NHS rationing. After the Collier case, however, the courts were to become more active.

Judicial activism

Jaymee Bowen's case (Girl B)

In 1995, the case of Girl B was brought first to the High Court and then to the Court of Appeal. Her clinical merits were less favourable than those of little boy Collier. She had a poorly responding leukaemia, the proposed treatment was experimental and debilitating, and was estimated to cost £75,000. On the responsible doctor's advice, Cambridge and Huntingdon Health Authority refused to support the treatment and her father made an application for judicial review. Significantly, the High Court overturned the decision to refuse treatment and referred it back to the authority to be reconsidered. It said that, in a case involving the life of a child, the authority must do more than 'toll the bell of scarce resources'. This resonating phrase seems to have signalled a dramatic change in judicial attitude. Although the case was taken to the Court of Appeal where the decision of the health authority was affirmed, subsequent cases have taken a more critical view of decisions to deny patients access to treatment. Note that, unlike Collier, the responsible doctors in Girl B did not consider further treatment to be in her best interests.

The 'transsexuals' case (A, D & G)

In A, D & G, three patients suffered gender identity dysphoria and requested transsexual surgery. Their request was refused by the health authority. Application for judicial review was made to the Court of Appeal. Consistent with Hincks, the judges confirmed that rationing was not unlawful in principle. It was lawful, therefore, for health authorities to construct a priority framework and to put transsexual surgery low on the list of priorities. Significantly, however, it said that the process of rationing has to be fair, consistent and reasonable. The process used in this case failed to meet these requirements because it failed to consider whether these individuals had exceptional needs for the treatment. The application for judicial review was successful and the health authority's refusal was referred back to be reconsidered. The case shows that economics can facilitate the creation of general policies, but those policies must allow for the possibility of exceptional claims arising which are considered on their own individual merits.

Rationing at health authority level

We have seen how rationing is lawful in principle. With the separation of purchaser and provider functions, responsibility for resource allocation in secondary care moved to the health authorities. However, as the transsexual case demonstrates, the emphasis was on the process by which rationing occurs. The next question, therefore, is how should rationing take place. The case of A, D & G discusses the procedures for deciding which treatments will and will not be provided. Any such process must be fair, and reasonably consistent between patients. This demands a clear and coherent policy which probably requires the creation of a reliable committee made up of well informed people with a cross-section of relevant interests – for example managers, doctors, nurses and patients representatives. It is not a function for a single person. What factors should such a committee consider? The court said it should carefully assess:

- the nature and seriousness of each type of illness
- the various forms of treatment for it
- any exceptional 'needs' of individual patients.

In addition, it would also be reasonable to consider the cost of treatment relative to other treatments. Finally, the policy should be applied fairly and consistently between patients.

Thus, priorities committees should devise a general framework of values (which may differ from place to place). However, allowance must be made for exceptional cases. This means that 'blanket bans' on treatment are unacceptable. This is because all the relevant factors should be considered, one of which must be any exceptional circumstances which are special to particular patients. Even patients low on the priorities framework should be given the opportunity to explain why they consider their needs to be exceptional. As we have seen, this means that an economic analysis may well be relevant in the formulation of the coherent priorities policy, but it cannot be used as the only yardstick of entitlement. Procedures for considering exceptional cases must also exist. They are not supposed to be 'legalised' so that they resemble a court hearing with examination and cross-examination of witnesses. Patients should be able to put a special case in writing before the authority and the case should be reconsidered in a way that is independent of the original decision. The patient must be given sufficient information about the reasons for the refusal to enable him or her to make a reasoned response. Such a committee should keep a record of the cases it hears and of the numbers that succeed and fail. Otherwise, it might appear that it is has not properly considered the merits of the case and is really a rubber stamp.

Rationing at the national level: 'guidance', 'directions' and the status of NICE

With resource decisions taken at health authority level, it was inevitable that there would be non-uniformity in both the process of decision making and the decisions that were taken. The inevitable result was 'postcode rationing' which was seen as unacceptable in a national health service. In April 1999, the National Institute for Clinical Excellence (NICE) was set up to 'enable evidence of clinical and cost effectiveness to be integrated to inform a national judgement on the value of a treatment(s) relative to alternative uses of the resources' and thereby provide 'guidance on whether a treatment (new or existing) can be recommended for routine use in the NHS (in England and Wales)'. Until recently, NICE's recommendations were guidance only (Box 23.1). As such, they had to be conscientiously taken into account by priorities committees, but it was not binding upon them.

However, from 2002, NICE guidance has the status of directions. The difference between mere 'guidance' and 'directions' is that directions are binding.

Box 23.1:   The nature of guidance

The legal authority of guidance is demonstrated in the case of Fisher in 1997. The Secretary of State published guidance recommending the use of beta-interferon for those suffering multiple sclerosis. North Derbyshire Health Authority did not wish to implement the guidance. In judicial review proceedings brought by an aggrieved patient, the court decided that the authority had introduced a blanket ban on beta-interferon. This was held to be irrational. Such a policy failed to include national policy (expressed in the guidance) as a relevant consideration in its decision making. As the transsexuals' case demonstrates, the authority were entitled to manage their own priorities policy. However, the condition had to be placed somewhere in their framework of priorities, and allowance had to be made for 'exceptional cases'.

The National Health Service Act 1977 gives them mandatory force. This means that those to whom they are directed are obliged to adhere to them. What do the NICE directions mandate? Before they were published, they were promoted by the DoH as providing patients with a 'guarantee' of access to care recommended by NICE, provided their doctors prescribed it. However, the wording of the direction itself is much less clear. The direction says that within three months of NICE guidance, 'A Health Authority shall . . . apply such amounts paid to it . . . as may be required so as to ensure that a [treatment] recommended by the Institute . . . is normally available . . .'

What is meant by 'normally available'? The Direction provides a presumption that NICE guidance will be funded unless there are persuasive reasons why it should not. For example, NICE does not affect the duty of PCTs to live within the annual budgets (*see* s 97, National Health Service Act 1977). Thus, if an authority could demonstrate that the guidance could not be accommodated until additional funds became available, this might be lawful. For example, some guidance may require substantial investment in training, or additional staff, or facilities. Such an investment might not be normally available within 3 months. Also, it would probably be lawful to advise against use of treatment which reasonable and reliable evidence indicated was unsafe, or inappropriate for particular patients. Indeed, there might be a duty to issue such advice.

Of course, doctors still retain their normal clinical discretion. The NICE direction places no obligation to prescribe because its guidance is intended to benefit aggregates of population – it could never be perfect for each individual patient. So the doctor must retain the freedom to decide for whom it will, and will not, be beneficial.

Rationing in primary care

We have seen that NHS rationing is lawful. In principle, therefore, it could also be lawful in primary care. However, rationing in primary care is covered by an entirely different set of rights and obligations. It is different because GPs are governed by separate rules under the General Medical Services (GMS) and Personal Medical Services (PMS) regulations, by which Parliament imposes special rights and obligations. Here, we consider the GP's GMS and PMS duties and the position of non-GP prescribers.

The duty of GPs to prescribe under GMS

Unlike hospital doctors under contracts of employment, GPs are governed by their GMS Terms of Service with PCTs. This is a statutory contract imposed by Parliament under the National Health Service Act 1977. It also means that GPs cannot pick and choose from the various rights and duties it contains. The GP's Terms of Service were first introduced by Secretary of State Nye Bevan in 1948 – they have a pedigree! They also make rationing in primary care difficult to accommodate in law. This may sound perverse. Why should there be a profound difference between secondary care (where rationing is permitted) and primary care (where, it seems, it is not)? This is the significance of the historical pedigree because 'enshrined' rights in the NHS are difficult to change. In brief, prescribing rights are contained in paragraphs 12 and 43 of the Terms of Service (Box 23.2).

Notice the use of the word 'shall'. This is very different from 'may', or 'shall within available resources'. What effect do these provisions have on the duty to prescribe? Patient 'need' must depend on a reasonable clinical assessment

---

Box 23.2:   Prescribing rights contained in the GP's Terms of Service

Paragraph 12(1) provides: 'A doctor shall render to his patients all necessary and appropriate personal medical services of the type usually provided by general practitioners.' This includes '... arranging for the referral of patients, as appropriate, for the provision of any other services under the Act ... (para.12(2)(d)).' And paragraph 43 requires that, subject to products on the 'black' and 'grey' lists, 'a doctor shall order any drugs or appliances which are needed for the treatment of any patient to whom he is providing treatment under these terms of service by issuing to that patient a prescription form.'

by the responsible GP. The terms of service do not require doctors to prescribe anything patients want – indeed, that could be dangerous and negligent. Also unexplained prescribing variations between doctors need addressing. For this reason, pharmacists are playing an important role assisting and advising doctors. GPs must take their advice and guidance seriously. Wasteful prescribing can be punished by deductions from the GP's remuneration (see the Service and Committee Tribunal Regs). In extreme cases, the doctor may be removed from the medical list (s 25, Health and Social Care Act 2001). All this is reasonable and proper. However, what about responsible prescribing that is expensive and will exceed the target budget?

Two things suggest that the duty to prescribe is not cash limited and the duty to prescribe is dependent on the responsible doctor's assessment of each patient's individual needs. The first comes from the NHSE. While urging GPs to live within their budgets Developing Primary Care Groups (HSC 1998/139, paras. 52–53) advises that 'The new system will continue to allow individual GPs to decide what is best for the patient, whether for example, to prescribe drugs or refer patients to hospital on the basis of their clinical judgement. The freedom to refer and prescribe remains unchanged. Patients will continue to be guaranteed the drugs, investigations and treatments they need. There will be no question of anyone being denied the drugs they need because the GP or Primary Care Group have run out of cash. GPs' participation in a primary care group will not affect their ability to fulfil their terms of service obligation always to prescribe and refer in the best interest of their patients.'

The second factor is the case of Pfizer, (the 'Viagra' case), the only decision on the Terms of Service duty to prescribe. Soon after 'Viagra' received its licence, the Secretary of State decided to include it on the 'grey' list for restricted use. However, this process requires Parliamentary time and, pending its inclusion on the list, he told GPs not to prescribe it except in limited cases. This interim guidance was held to be unlawful. The High Court held, with reference to paragraphs 12 and 43, '. . . The doctor must give such treatment as he, exercising the professional judgment to be expected from an average GP, considers necessary and appropriate . . .' The guidance in question trespassed on the proper statutory responsibilities imposed on GPs by the GMS regulations. It would have been permissible for the Secretary of State to urge doctors to be cautious, 'but [he] must make it clear that the GP's clinical judgment is supreme'.

Presumably, this applies equally to treatments which NICE have not recommended. Thus, paragraphs 12 and 43 of the Terms of Service seem to impose a duty on the GP to prescribe on the basis of need which does not accommodate resource constraints. Of course, drugs can be placed on the 'black' and 'grey' lists (like Viagra). Until then, the Terms of Service appear to make rationing very difficult in primary care. Clearly, the Terms of Service make the cost management of responsible prescribing very difficult. Within the constraints of a fixed PCT budget, it has serious implications for the sums available elsewhere.

The duty of GPs to prescribe under PMS

What about PMS doctors? The short answer is that their position is identical to their GMS colleagues. The PMS directions, which form the foundation for all the agreements made under the scheme says, 'Where any drugs, medicines or listed appliances are needed for the treatment of any patient paragraphs 43 to 46 of Schedule 2 to the GMS Regulations shall apply' (para. 2, sched. 1). The opportunity to introduce a power to ration within PMS was not taken (perhaps for fear of reintroducing a 'two-tier' system of access to care). Exactly why such a radically different approach should be taken to NHS rationing in primary care by comparison to secondary care has never been explained. Clearly, these duties to treat on the basis of individual need contradict principles of health economics which are concerned with identifying opportunity costs and benefits to populations as a whole.

Non-GP prescribers

What about the prescribing rights of non-GP prescribers? Nurses and pharmacists, for example, have had their prescribing rights extended. Their position is different because they are not subject to the Terms of Service. They are employees subject to a contract of employment. Nevertheless, when a GP engages others to work for him or her who are not on the medical list, the GP's duties under the Terms of Service remain intact. The GP is 'responsible for all the acts and omissions of ... any person employed by ... him' (GP's Terms of Service, para. 20). Were the GP to employ someone on terms which prevented the employee from fulfilling the obligations imposed upon the GP, the GP himself, or herself, could be in breach of his/her terms of service.

On the other hand, PCTs may also employ non-GP prescribing staff in this way who are not subject to the Terms of Service. If staff were employed on terms that required them to ration treatment which was needed, this could lead to a different quality of service. The danger of a 'two-tier' service might resurface so that patients would want to know whether their 'prescriber' was acting under the Terms of Service or as a PCT employee.

Conclusion

We started by asking how law affects rationing in the NHS and whether an economic analysis provides answers. In secondary care, we saw that since

1997 (with the case of Fisher) the law has had a significant impact on NHS resource allocation. In particular, as the case of the 'transsexuals' shows, well-informed rationing policies are essential to a fair and consistent approach between competing demands. However, they must also allow for the possibility that patients who find themselves low on the priorities list may have exceptional circumstances which deserve treatment. Therefore, the policy must enable patients access to an exceptional review of their case. Blanket bans are not acceptable.

In primary care, we noted the extraordinary Terms of Service promise, first made in 1948, that GPs should treat patients on the basis of need. Unlike the duty in secondary care which is based on proper processes, the Terms of Service promises treatment. New Terms of Service are expected in 2002. Within the constraints of funding, perhaps it is time to consider introducing rationing in primary care too. However, if we do so let us also exhort government to involve itself, for once, in the debate as to the care that patients should expect within the NHS, and what should be excluded.

Within this legal framework, therefore, economic analyses to healthcare do not fit the model very well. True, blanket approaches to care based on opportunity costs are entirely logical at one level. However, the judges suggest that they pay insufficient regard to the exceptional needs of individuals. Economics also sits very uncomfortably with the GP's Terms of Service obligation to treat on the basis of need.

Space does not permit extended discussion of the Human Rights Act 1998.[1] Other than in wholly exceptional circumstances, however, the European Convention is unlikely to confer 'positive' rights on individuals (i.e. giving rights to resources). It is more comfortable in the field of 'negative' rights (i.e. protection from interference). For this reason, it is unlikely to demand that nation states commit a certain proportion of their gross domestic product to health, education, the environment and so on. It has no expertise to do so; and, in any case, this is a matter for the democratic process.

Regulations and cases

NHS (General Medical Services) Regulations 1992/635, as amended.
National Health Service (Service Committees and Tribunal) Regulations (1992) S.I. no. 644, reg. 15(1) and paras. 15 and 16.
R v Central Birmingham Health Authority, ex p Collier (Court of Appeal, 1988, unreported).
R v Cambridge and Huntingdon Health Authority, ex p Girl B (1995) 2 All England Law Reports 129.
R v NW Lancashire Health Authority, ex p A, D & G (2000) 53 Butterworths Medico Legal Reports 148.

R v North Berbyshire Health Authority, ex p Fisher (1997) 8 Medical Law Reports 327.
R v Secretary of State v Hincks (decided in 1980) (1992) Butterworths Medico Legal Reports 93.
R v Secretary of State, ex p Pfizer (1999) Lloyd's Reports Medical 289.

Reference

1   Lilley R, Lambden P and Newdick C (2001) *Understanding the Human Rights Act.* Radcliffe Medical Press, Oxford, 79–88.

Section 6

Health economics: some perspectives

Anyone who has managed to get this far in the book will have realised that there are a number of concerns with health economic theory and its application to resource allocation decisions. We all operate within our individual paradigms – the models with which we look at the world to describe what is happening. These conceptual frameworks are influenced and consolidated by our professional associations and the language that we use which in turn dictates the way that we explore, analyse and act. This final section offers a series of perspectives on health economics through different conceptual lenses.

Joanna Coast starts by expanding on the fundamental methodology and philosophy of health economics and how the discipline is adapting to reflect a less than perfect world. We then move on to some pragmatic concerns. Denis Pereira Gray, former President of the Royal College of General Practitioners, offers a view from his profession arguing that there are difficulties in undertaking economic analyses in this area due to the problems of identifying and quantifying its outputs.

From the broader perspective of the health authority, Gill Morgan describes the difficulties of decision making in an environment of multiple constraints, conflicting values and limited room for manoeuvre, and suggests that we should be happy as ugly ducklings, not swans.

We then continue with a more theoretical discourse. Donald Light offers the sociologist's viewpoint, arguing that much of what we do in healthcare takes place within a socially negotiated framework that is shaped by institutions, culture, history and power; factors that are invariably overlooked by a purely economic approach. Paul Webley considers the neglect of psychology by health economics and suggests that marrying the top-down approach of economics with the bottom-up insights of psychologists may lead to a more applicable and usable discipline. The philosophical lens comes next although I am never quite sure what philosophers do. My suspicion is that they study how language forms a metaphorical bridge to reality. When I asked Martyn Evans, who contributes this chapter, he clarified my thinking by advising me that a philosopher is someone for whom the questions we ask in the pub on Friday night are still real on Monday afternoon when sober.

Chapter 30 carries a health warning for economists. From the perspective of the healthcare practitioner, the fact that nature does not divide itself up into neat divisions such as economics, sociology and psychology seems to have been conveniently overlooked. These divisions are imposed upon her by historical processes that are codified and consolidated in ivory towers, detached from the contingencies of the real world. I briefly describe how the emerging field of complexity theory can offer an overarching perspective or 'meta view' of healthcare organisation, yielding important insights into the decision-making processes within it.

I extend the courtesy of the last word to Alan Maynard who, in a storming rear guard action, argues that despite all criticisms the health economic tribe will not go away.

CHAPTER 24

The philosophical and methodological basis of health economics

Joanna Coast

Economic theory can be used to try to explain and predict how health-care systems work. This chapter explores the basic principles upon which economic theory is based and how these principles can be applied to health-care. In applying mainstream economics to health and healthcare, health economists have, inevitably, become aware of some of the limitations of these theories compared with the realities of healthcare provision.

Key points
- Philosophy and method in health economics are largely based on the two branches of mainstream economics.
- The first (positive or explanatory economics) uses assumptions about how consumers (patients) and firms (healthcare providers including doctors and hospitals) act, to develop explanations and predictions about the operation of healthcare systems.
- The second (normative or welfare economics) aims to develop empirical evidence for choosing healthcare interventions on the grounds of max-imising the total benefit available from limited healthcare resources.
- In some areas, developments in health economics are challenging the mainstream philosophy and method.

Chapter sections
- **Introduction**
- **Using economic theory to obtain knowledge**
- **Using economic theory to make decisions**
- **Developments in health economics**
- **Conclusion**

Introduction

It is standard to consider health economics as the discipline of economics applied to the topic of health. Both the philosophical and methodological bases of health economics are, as a result, founded on their similar bases in economics. Economics, like the other social sciences, has developed its own particular way of looking at the world. Whereas sociology focuses on social interaction and the relationships, such as power, within that interaction, and psychology focuses on the individual, economics is concerned with the allocation of scarce resources and, particularly, with the operation of market mechanisms.

There are two distinct branches of economics, and this distinction carries through into health economics. The first branch of economics tries to use theory to explain and predict the operation of the economic system. This is sometimes referred to as positive or explanatory economics. The second branch of economics assumes particular values and then tries to go about achieving those. This is sometimes referred to as normative or welfare economics. Economists working within these two branches are essentially trying to achieve different things – the first group is concerned with obtaining knowledge, the second with making decisions. These two different aspects of economics are discussed below. The final part of the chapter describes some of the recent concerns of health economists in terms of philosophy and methodology, and some of the changes that they have been making.

Using economic theory to obtain knowledge

Economic theory can be used to try to explain and predict how healthcare systems work. In trying to do this, health economists generally start from a particular view of the world, based on the mainstream economic view. (Although mainstream economics does not reach back so far, Mill's 1836 essay 'On the definition of political economy and the method of investigation proper to it'[1] provides a basic explanation of method as it is still largely understood in economics.) At the simplest level, economists tend to think about the world as being divided into consumers and firms. In terms of healthcare, consumers would be patients, and firms would include all those involved in producing healthcare: hospitals, general practices, doctors and so on.

In this view of the world, firms are assumed to be motivated by profit and consumers are assumed to be self-interested and to act rationally so as to maximise their utility. Utility is a term used by economists to describe consumer preferences (Box 24.1); an alternative way of thinking about it is in terms of satisfaction or happiness.

Box 24.1:   The concept of utility

In the nineteenth century, economists tended to think of utility as something that could be measured cardinally (that is, like length, where the numbers attached to utility have some significance). Such cardinal measurement would imply that it is possible to compare utility across individuals. In the twentieth century, economists have generally made this assumption less restrictive by accepting that interpersonal comparison of utility is impossible, and assuming only that utility is ordinal (that is, that consumers can rank according to preference, but that numbers attached to utility have no meaning beyond this ability to rank). However measured, utility is a number representing the preference for a particular bundle of goods or services.

Basic building blocks of positive economics

Consumers' preferences are also believed to conform to certain assumptions.

- They are assumed to be complete, in that all goods and services can be compared.
- They are assumed to be reflexive, in that if one good is identical to another good, the preference for it will be at least as high.
- They are assumed to be transitive, in that if a person prefers apples to oranges, and oranges to pears, then they will prefer apples to pears.
- Most importantly, perhaps, consumers are assumed to know what their preferences are.

Economists use these basic assumptions (or axioms) as the building blocks for developing theory. They are looking to find a set of laws which can explain a single, and potentially knowable, reality. To these basic axioms, others are added to develop a theory about a particular aspect of the economy. Hypotheses are developed from this theory and are then tested quantitatively to determine whether the theory should be accepted or rejected.

Problems with applying economic axioms to healthcare

Applying the basic axioms to healthcare is, however, problematic. Certain of these assumptions do not hold where health is concerned. In particular, 'firms' providing healthcare do not tend to be motivated by profit: doctors tend to be motivated by caring for the individual patient and there are codes of ethics which govern their practice; managers may be motivated by the size of their department. Consumers, on the other hand, may well be motivated by maximising their utility – but do not have the expertise to fully know their preferences. Thus the theories have been adapted to try to account for these sorts of problems, for example, by looking at how patients use doctors as an 'agent' to help make decisions on their behalf – the doctor provides the expertise that the patient does not have and helps the patient to make a decision that maximises the patient's preferences. In turn, however, this notion of an 'agency-relationship' suggests further problems with how the healthcare system works because doctors acting on behalf of the patient may have an incentive to follow their own preferences (for increased salary, or for more interesting work) rather than strictly those of the patient. In practice, many of the economic theories surrounding healthcare are concerned with this sort of problem, of why the healthcare 'market' does not work in the same way as other markets in the economy. The hope is that, by understanding better how healthcare systems work, it becomes possible to develop methods of overcoming some of the problems.

Using economic theory to make decisions

Economics can also be used to try to improve how decisions are made about which interventions to pursue. This branch of economics, welfare economics, began to develop around the turn of the twentieth century, and is concerned with how to allocate resources optimally. Again, economists have started from a small number of very basic assumptions in developing theory about how decisions can be improved.

Basic building blocks for normative economics

Three assumptions in particular are important and form the building blocks for the assessment of efficiency, where efficiency is defined as 'ensuring that goods and services are allocated so as to maximise the welfare of the community'.[2]

- Individuals are the best judges of their own welfare (welfare can be seen as depending both on the individual's utility and their view of the distribution of well-being among all members of a community).[3]

- A movement to a state where one individual can be made better off without any other individual being made worse off can be seen as an improvement in social welfare.
- More controversial is that a movement to a particular state can also be seen as beneficial if the individual(s) gaining from that move could, potentially, compensate those who lose – although such compensation would not have to be paid in practice.

The importance of the third assumption in making the leap to this definition of efficiency is often overlooked. What the third assumption does, is to allow economists to abstract from issues of the distribution of resources in making statements about 'more' and 'less' efficient uses of resources. Of course, however, this abstraction may be particularly problematic in healthcare, given that compensating people for death and even for severely reduced health states would be impossible. Health economists are well aware of these problems, but the difficulty is, that without some value judgements, it is difficult to make any statement about how to make choices between alternatives.

Efficiency and economic evaluation

The practical expression of this search for efficiency in healthcare is the conduct of economic evaluation. This is a catch-all term for the various methods of measuring and comparing the costs and benefits of different healthcare interventions and has been discussed fully in Chapter 3. The aim is to work out how to maximise the benefit available from the limited resources for healthcare. Methodology here is based very much on the empirical estimation of these costs and benefits, and economists work closely with epidemiologists and statisticians to ensure that costs are measured in an unbiased fashion alongside randomised trials comparing the effectiveness of interventions. They also work closely with psychologists and qualitative researchers to develop instruments that can measure the benefits of healthcare accurately in a manner which is useful for making statements about relative costs and benefits.

Developments in health economics

In applying mainstream economics to health and healthcare, health economists have, inevitably, become aware of some of the limitations of these theories compared with the realities of healthcare provision. This final part of the chapter looks at three of the recent concerns of health economists, and how they are addressing them.

First, as in mainstream economics, some health economists have noted that there are problems in developing explanations on the basis of assumptions about how people behave rather than observations of how they actually behave in practice. A number of health economists have started to use qualitative methods in their work to attempt to develop theory inductively,[4,5] that is, on the basis of observing institutions and systems, and talking to the people involved about their views and perceptions. Such work has concentrated on how decisions about contracts and priority setting actually happen in practice, and in determining the influences on these decisions.[6]

Second, economists working on the decision-making aspect of health economics have noted that the efficiency findings of economic evaluations are not necessarily taken account of by decision makers, and have concluded that this is because the value system of society does not necessarily accord with that currently understood by economists. Health economists have done a lot of work in recent years, both quantitative and qualitative, to try to find out more about what citizens and health professionals feel are the values which should inform how decisions are made in healthcare (for example, see the work by Nord et al.,[7,8] Ubel,[9] and Dolan et al.[10]). As a result, much greater attention is now being paid by health economists to issues of equity and distribution.

Third, some health economists have formed the view that, in respect of healthcare, patients (consumers) may not be the best judge of their own welfare, and that the aim of the healthcare system is not to maximise consumer welfare, but instead to maximise health (on the basis that this is what decision makers see as their objective). Health economists taking this sort of view have become known as 'extra-welfarist'[11] and have provided the spur for the development of health status measures that produce a single value for the gain in health as a result of an intervention.

Conclusion

The philosophy and methodology of health economics is largely associated with that of mainstream economics. As a result it is, for the most part, based on the view that knowledge is obtained by developing theory based on a number of assumptions, testing these theories and choosing to accept or reject them on the basis of the evidence obtained. Nevertheless, these philosophies and methods are not set in stone. Many of the theories and methods of mainstream economics have served health economists well in the past in providing insight into the operation of healthcare systems, and they will continue to do so in the future. Yet there are also limitations. Health economists are concerned with how decisions are made in practice and in improving the ability of the work produced by health economists to assist in this decision making. Where current philosophies and methods appear to be failing health economists in dealing with the realities of healthcare, there are changes taking place to the established methods. Health economics is a young and dynamic subdiscipline of economics, drawing on mainstream economics where this serves it best, but adapting and changing to develop theory which also allows for the realities of healthcare provision.

References

1   Mill JS (1994) On the definition and method of political economy. In: DM Hausman (ed) *The Philosophy of Economics: an anthology*. Cambridge University Press, Cambridge, 52–68.

2   Drummond MF (1991) Output measurement for resource-allocation decisions in healthcare. In: A McGuire (ed) *Providing Health Care: the economics of alternative systems of finance and delivery*. Oxford University Press, Oxford, 99–119.

3   Scitovsky T (1951) The state of welfare economics. *Am Economic Rev.* **41**: 303–15.

4   Coast J (2001) Citizens, their agents and healthcare rationing: an exploratory study using qualitative methods. *Health Economics.* **10**: 159–74.

5   Goddard M, Mannion R and Smith P (2000) Enhancing performance in healthcare: a theoretical perspective on agency and the role of information. *Health Economics.* **9**: 95–107.

6   Mannion R and Smith P (1997) Trust and reputation in community care. In: P Anand (ed) *Changes in Health Care: reflections on the NHS internal market*. MacMillan, Basingstoke, 141–61.

7   Nord E, Richardson J, Street A, Kuhse H and Singer P (1995) Who cares about cost? Does economic analysis impose or reflect social values? *Health Policy.* **34**: 79–94.

8   Nord E (1993) The relevance of health state after treatment in prioritising between different patients. *J Med Ethics.* **19**: 37–42.

9   Ubel PA (1999) How stable are people's preferences for giving priority to severely ill patients? *Soc Sci Med.* **49**: 895–903.

10 Dolan P and Cookson R (2000) A qualitative study of the extent to which health gain matters when choosing between groups of patients. *Health Policy.* **51**: 19–30.

11 Culyer AJ (1989) The normative economics of health care finance and provision. *Oxford Rev Econ Pol.* **5**: 34–56.

CHAPTER 25

Economic evaluation and general practice

Denis Pereira Gray

Introduction

The principles of health economics are well known, but their application to general medical practice is relatively new. General practice holds the central place in the NHS in the United Kingdom and it is helpful and timely to start discussions now for a number of reasons.

First, 97% of the whole population is registered with the NHS, making it the most widely used public service. General practitioners are the largest branch of the medical profession.

Second, they have the largest contacts of any group of doctors with the population as a whole. The contact rate is so great that there were 269 million consultations between patients and their general practitioners in 1998.[1]

Third, the scale of activity has major impacts on other parts of the NHS. The vast majority of the costs of pharmaceuticals in the NHS flow from general practitioner decisions and prescriptions. For example, the average number of prescriptions written by general practitioners per patient in the NHS is now as high as 11 per year (Department of Health, personal communication). The great majority of admissions to hospital are as a result of referrals by general practitioners, who are therefore one of the key drivers of all costs in the NHS as a whole. Furthermore, it is not just a matter of money, but of life and death; Jarman *et al.* showed that the death rate of patients in British hospitals inversely correlated with the number of general practitioners in the surrounding community.[2] Doctors who had fewer patients in some way judged admissions better, that is, to their patients' advantage.

Health economists offer insights into the operation of general practice from both the positive (descriptive) and normative (prescriptive) perspectives. This chapter focuses on the latter framework which is known as economic analysis – a technique that relates the benefits of an intervention to the resources used in their production. With the emphasis on a primary care led NHS and the development of skill mix, this exercise is becoming increasingly important for the general practitioner. The consultation forms the core of general practice activity and the cost of a consultation is well defined.[3] The big question is that of the value of the outputs of general practice, but there are great difficulties in answering the question. This chapter outlines some of those difficulties as a means of fostering further research on the subject.

The outputs from general practice

In many economic activities such as manufacturing, costs of all the inputs such as raw materials, staff and equipment are well defined. The output they produce is easily identified and has a market price. In general practice the outputs are not well defined, and the important question is 'what are the outputs of this activity and the value placed on them'?

Making diagnoses

One key role for doctors in the front line of a national health system is the process of making diagnoses. Most diagnoses are made in general practice – the *General Household Survey*[4] shows that of all the problems people bring to the service, 86% are managed entirely in general practice/primary care and only 14% are referred to hospital.

Taking a common chronic disease like hypertension, which can affect up to 10% of the population, there must be a value in making the diagnosis. However, it is not immediately clear what this value is. Unfortunately, even after the diagnosis is made substantial proportions of patients either do not get, or get but do not take, the appropriate treatment. Only a minority of patients achieve control to levels shown by the research literature to be optimal.[5]

The value of an agreed output of controlled hypertension is easier to make. The proportion of uncontrolled patients who go on to suffer strokes is known, hence the number of strokes prevented can be calculated and the value of such an activity costed once a value of not having a stroke is agreed.

Similarly, in a screening programme, say cervical cytology, it is easier to calculate the value by concentrating on the minority of women who are identified as positive. It can then be calculated approximately how many could be expected to progress to cervical cancer and how much each case prevented is worth.

Management of chronic diseases

Many chronic diseases carry the risk of premature death, and/or complications reducing the quality of life. To clarify the value of good primary care it will be necessary to place a value on a life lost or lost earlier than the usual expectation of life. This is distasteful for doctors who are not yet accustomed to think in these terms, but such thinking is common, indeed usual in other fields.

For example, the Department of Transport decides whether or not to undertake road improvements on the basis of the average number of deaths the improvement is expected to save. This leads to the need to place a cash value on a human life. It is interesting that, outside healthcare, this value in 2000 is about one million pounds. In medical care lives can be saved much more cheaply. For example, the Wanless Report shows that a life year can be gained by the use of statins in the secondary prevention of ischaemic heart disease for as little as £4000.[6] Bunker and colleagues have approached the question of the value of medical care in a broader but similar way, and have concluded that modern medicine has been undervalued in its effectiveness.[7,8]

They counter the original conclusion of McKeown, in his Rock Carling Lecture, that the main causes of lives gained have been through environmental reforms such as clean water and air.[9] Bunker and colleagues believe that as these environmental factors are increasingly improved, the contribution of modern medicine becomes more important. They suggest that about half the gains in life expectancy are now due to medical care. This condenses down to the fact that often more lives can be saved in health for a given expenditure than in many other forms of public spending.

Thus in determining the value of, say, a general practice with 150 diabetic patients, it would be necessary to measure how well the disease was controlled and then calculate the death rate expected and the complication rate expected for such a population. Finally, it is necessary to put a value on each life and complication. One day all this will be done.

Reassurance

Reassurance is a core activity of all primary care services, but it is surprisingly difficult to identify and value. First, there is the simple issue of coding general practice consultations in which the endpoint is reassurance. If a patient visits the doctor with say palpitations, but really fears he is going to have a heart attack, then reassurance as the output may be lost in symptomatic recording as, say, 'palpitations'. Similarly, a patient presenting with a headache, who really fears that she has a brain tumour may be recorded in the computer records as 'headache'. Such problems are not easily retrieved from most general practice computer systems. Worse still, when recorded, the activities are divided among all the various symptom complexes in different systems of the body.

This means that it is quite hard to measure even the frequency of significant reassurance, let alone its economic value. I have had patients coming into the consulting room shaking with fear, and going out laughing, a highly valuable consultation to the patient and to society. Yet my records often only categorised the consultation under some symptom heading. To the outside observer, general practice is thus consistently trivialised and hence devalued. This will continue until some way of separately recording the process of providing important reassurance, and probably classifying its importance to the patient, is introduced.

Support, empowerment, enablement

Vast numbers of people go to the doctor because they feel generally unwell or uneasy. A front line medical service seeing the whole population on average as often as four times a year has to be flexible and efficient.[4] It has to diagnose a life-threatening disease like meningitis from among a mass of similar flu-like conditions; it has to manage 90% of infections in all parts of the body; manage most of the common chronic diseases; and it has to provide support, encouragement and, if possible, empowerment to most of these patients. Howie and his colleagues have been among the first to measure this role which they called 'enablement'.[10] This is a term describing how most people seeing an NHS general practitioner within the constraints of the service felt better able to cope with whatever problem they had. This may be one interesting overall summary statistic for the general practice service, but it remains for others to cost its value to patients and society.

The value of human relationships

The human side of medicine alters the dynamics and affects outcomes in many ways. Thus continuity of primary care has been shown to be associated with the development of trust in the doctor by the patient. Simultaneously, Charney *et al.* and Ettlinger and Freeman have shown that the willingness of patients to take the medication prescribed, is affected by how much they trust the doctor.[11,12] Gill and Mainous have shown that continuity of primary care is associated with a reduction in future hospital admissions.[13]

In health economic terms these findings complicate the measurement of value. A series of consultations with the same doctor become more valuable than the same number of consultations with different doctors, as the continuity achieved has a separate value over and above the care provided in each individual consultation. This too is not easy to extract from primary care records, and this absence again tends to undervalue primary care. Trust by patients in doctors can now be measured and is associated with continuity of care.[14]

Seeing two or more patients at once

The importance of family doctors seeing two or more patients in a single consultation has been noted and valued.[15] Yet this is so common to appear not worth recording, nor is it usually recorded, even in consultations in general practice in the year 2001. Yet small children are virtually always accompanied to the doctor. Consultations about the child are recorded in the child's record. The parent may do most of the talking and ask all the key questions. The answers, if recorded at all, are in the child's record. The doctor after several such consultations may learn a great deal about say the mother's personality, and her hopes and fears. Her doctor may have gained great understanding about her as a person and her needs, albeit through the medium of her child, but this is often not recorded in her record and will not be valued under current systems of analysis.

Even when two people consult at once and when both medical records record the care provided, there are problems. For example, if a mother seeks contraceptive advice, say a repeat prescription for the pill during an appointment for child care surveillance, then both the child and mother's record will usually record the treatment and advice given. However, the appointment book, computerised or not, will show only a single consultation. When trying to relate inputs to outputs in such a practice, these highly efficient consultations where two quite separate problems were simultaneously resolved for two different people will be diminished. If general practice is ever disaggregated, so that different people do one or the other of these tasks, the 'extra work' will be revealed as extra consultations with extra costs.

Conclusion

The process of applying health economic analyses to general practice is in its infancy and faces larger problems than other activities such as surgical operations. Precisely because general practitioners are generalists, their outputs are multiple and less easy to quantify than in most branches of medicine.[16] The traditional system of record keeping needs review, and computers may open up for the first time a way of capturing more completely the diverse functions of doctors working in the front line of the NHS.[17] Some key functions like reassurance are almost lost in symptom recording. Multiple consultations and building up a deep understanding of patients as people are fundamental efficiency factors. They do not easily show and so are easily devalued. General practice records understate some of the most important activities of primary care. The true value of general practice is thus constantly being underestimated.

Acknowledgements

Mrs Joy Choules, of SaNDNet, for help with references. The Fetzer Institute, Michigan, USA has funded the Institute of General Practice to research the doctor–patient relationship.

References

1 Office of Health Economics (2000) *Compendium of Health Statistics* (12e). OHE, London, Section 4.20, 35.

2 Jarman B, Gault S, Alves B *et al.* (1999) Explaining differences in English hospital death rates using routinely collected data. *BMJ.* **318:** 1515–20.

3 Netten A and Curtis L (2000) *The Unit Costs of Health and Social Care Report.* PSSRU, University of Kent, Canterbury.

4 Office for National Statistics Social Survey Division (1998) *Living in Britain – results from the 1996 general household survey.* The Stationery Office, London.

5 Chief Medical Officer of the Department of Health (2001) *On the State of the Public Health: annual report.* DoH, London.

6 Wanless D (2001) *Securing our Future Health: taking a long-term view.* HM Treasury, London.

7 Bunker JP, Frazier HS and Mosteller F (1994) Improving health: measuring effects of medical care. *Milbank Quarterly.* **72(2):** 225–58.

8 Bunker J (2001) *Medicine Matters After All.* The Stationery Office for the Nuffield Trust, London.

9 McKeown T (1976) *The Role of Medicine. Dream, Mirage, or Nemesis?* Nuffield Provincial Hospitals Trust, London.

10 Howie JGR, Heaney DJ and Maxwell M (1997) *Measuring Quality in General Practice.* Occasional Paper 75. RCGP, Exeter.

11 Charney E, Bynum R and Eldridge DE (1967) How well do patients take oral penicillin? *Pediatrics.* **40:** 188–95.

12 Ettlinger PRA and Freeman GR (1981) General practice compliance study: is it worth being a doctor? *BMJ.* **282:** 1192–3.

13 Gill JM and Mainous AG (1998) The role of provider continuity in preventing hospitalizations. *Arch Fam Med.* **7:** 352–7.

14 Mainous AGI, Baker R, Love MM, Pereira Gray D and Gill JM (2001) Continuity of care and trust in one's physician: evidence from primary care in the United States and the United Kingdom. *Fam Med.* **33(1):** 22–7.

15 Pereira Gray DJ (1970) The care of the handicapped child in general practice: Gold Medal Essay 1969. *Transactions of the Hunterian Society.* **28:** 121–75.

16 Pereira Gray DJ, Steele R, Sweeney KG and Evans P (1994) Generalists in medicine (Editorial). *BMJ.* **308:** 486–7.

17 Royal College of General Practitioners (1987) *The Front Line of the Health Service.* Report from General Practice 25. RCGP, London.

CHAPTER 26

Being happy as ugly ducklings and not swans: the health authority perspective

Gill Morgan

Introduction

Health authorities manage and coordinate groups of organisations, which together make up a health community. They are charged with delivering governmental priorities by catalysing local action to improve health, reduce health inequalities, integrate services for patients and improve service quality. The broader health agenda requires close working and partnership with other agencies including social services, local government and the voluntary sector. Health services work to national standards identified in a series of National Service Frameworks, which cover a number of major health conditions. Delivery targets are set for a number of key issues, including waiting times and numbers of patients on waiting lists. Improvements to services are achieved by the effective commissioning of services by health authorities and primary care organisations. Shifting the balance of power will transfer most of these responsibilities to primary care trusts while the new strategic health authorities will become responsible for performance management, performance and capacity development and for ensuring delivery.

The problems for managers trying to deal with this complexity are acute. They need to reconcile central requirements with local needs and aspirations. In any system with a fixed budget, money or time spent on one area or service is at the expense of another (opportunity cost), and decisions need to take account of the impact of these lost opportunities as well as the benefits from any investment. The need to set priorities is thus a pervasive feature of all healthcare systems irrespective of the underlying level of funding. The choice between investments is more challenging in affluent societies where the relative differences in health benefit between potential areas of spend are usually marginal at best. The key question is whether a rational approach using health economic techniques can help us find a way through the complexities and politics of the healthcare system or whether health economics is merely 'nonsense on stilts'. This chapter reviews the difficulties of decision making in an environment of multiple constraints, conflicting values and limited room for manoeuvre.

The directives of historical precedent

Effective commissioning needs to recognise the particular health needs of the population served, understand the priorities of both national government and local communities, and appreciate the relative contribution and costs of the services needed to deliver the agreed outcomes. In a perfect world this would allow a comprehensive plan to be developed and delivered to meet assessed community needs. Health services have not, however, been developed in a rational way. Patterns of investment in every community reflect historical decisions and the relative power of different professional groups and organisations rather than being comprehensively and rationally planned to meet local health and healthcare needs. Health authorities work in a highly politicised environment with strong central direction and where there are many powerful vested interests competing for scarce resources at a local level. Existing incentive structures are geared towards the status quo and 'more of the same' rather than towards change and innovation. Precedent, tradition, power, rhetoric and media hype, together with professional self-interest, have therefore determined much of the service pattern seen in a community.

In the UK there has been a great deal of variability in service provision and significant local discretion since the inception of the NHS. While many differences have occurred by chance because of the political factors mentioned above, others reflect the different characteristics of the populations served including health status and geography. The patterns of service delivery and the healthcare needs of inner cities, for example, differ significantly from those of rural communities, and different service solutions have been identified to reflect this. While the many differences in services between communities is not discussed in the round, one aspect of this local sensitivity has generated significant debate. This is referred to as 'postcode prescribing' – that is the different availability of some expensive therapies and treatments between communities. This has been most highly publicised with beta-interferon for multiple sclerosis and with some expensive second and third in line cancer drugs, used when other therapies have failed. With the political wish to re-establish the NHS as a uniform service throughout the UK, postcode prescribing is now seen as unacceptable, and mechanisms have been put in place to ensure more uniform introduction of these therapies through the mandatory introduction of National Institute for

Clinical Excellence (NICE) recommendations. While superficially this seems laudable it does not take into account the local choices that have been made and the services that have been preferred in those communities that have rationed these expensive drugs.

Problems with conflicting values

Internationally, there have been a number of systematic attempts to use rational health economics based approaches for the allocation of resources. The initiatives in Oregon, the Netherlands and New Zealand are best known. None of the programmes have been as successful as was hoped in determining appropriate investment patterns. The approaches taken differ and are complex, but all have used a mixture of rational and value-based measures. Each model makes significant implicit judgements about how society values different health states, a key component of any comprehensive assessment of costs and benefits. This leaves them open to challenge. All similar approaches tend to value benefits for community (utilitarianism) over benefits for individuals (autonomy). This trade-off between community gain and individual capacity to benefit is at the heart of debates on priority setting. It is an increasingly difficult area for policy makers, with the growing focus on the rights of individuals now enshrined in human rights legislation. This legislation potentially conflicts with policies that emphasise the number of people likely to benefit from an intervention.

The problem is compounded by the difficulty of adequately and fairly assessing societal values. A number of different methods have been used to gauge these, often with uncomfortable results for policy makers. For example, treatment for drug addicts or alcoholics is frequently rated as being of low value to society because of the perceived personal responsibility and culpability of those affected. Advice about smoking cessation, the single most powerful public health intervention in terms of avoiding mortality and morbidity at very low cost, is often rated as low benefit as it crosses this line of perceived personal duty. Policy makers have been unable to handle this perceived perversity of societal values, and such aberrant results are either ignored or 'corrected' by eye to give them more face validity.

The other significant issue in healthcare is the role of clinical decision makers who have to balance the probability of success in a population with the potential for benefit of the individual they are treating. They wrestle with the fact that a therapy of low effectiveness in a population could have a very large potential benefit for an individual patient. Study design rarely identifies the factors that make a therapy successful for a particular sub-group of the population, and in many cases the response is personal and idiosyncratic. How can a clinician weigh these factors and make a rational decision when a patient is sitting across the desk? The evaluation of cancer drugs demonstrates this difficulty. Many of the new generation of drugs offer very little survival gain across the whole affected population, often at very high cost for a quality adjusted life year (QALY). Some of these drugs however, are reported as being so successful in some patients that tumour shrinkage occurs and curative resection becomes possible. The numbers needed to treat are large and prescription makes no sense at a population level, but at an individual level the benefits can be huge. How can this be factored into responsive and responsible decision making at a clinical level? It is much easier the further the decision is made from a patient where the needs for the population will swamp the benefits for an individual.

The fraught nature of this are highlighted by a number of high profile cases where individuals have fought health authorities in the press and in court for access to new therapies that they believe offer them the only chance of life. The health authorities concerned have made a rational estimate that the opportunity cost of introduction across the whole community is too large as, for the population as a whole, the therapy is not cost effective. Individuals and clinicians will always be biased towards overestimating the success of a therapy and looking for hope of success where the alternative is death or deterioration. The Americans call this the 'malignant optimism of oncologists'. It is, however, a perfectly rational and human response to the situation, and highlights the problem for methodologies which are scientific and do not recognise the fact that they are implemented by people with prejudices, vested interests and a strong sense of self preservation.

Practical problems in applying health economics

A further significant factor is the lack of available evidence about the cost benefit of new and, even more significantly, current therapies. Cost effectiveness of therapies is a key component of the assessment by NICE. The quality of the available evidence is, however, often extremely poor and based on manufacturer submissions and their economic models. These can be very complex and frequently, as might be anticipated, optimistic assumptions in key variables are made thus tending to underestimate the true cost per QALY. Much more emphasis on cost effectiveness is needed during the evaluation of new therapies. At a local level, however, even improved research on new therapies will be inadequate, as to make rational choices for a population based on cost effectiveness measures would require information about all the potential choices and the cost effectiveness and marginal benefits of each of these choices. We are light years away from having this amount of information or the skills to apply it appropriately in every healthcare system.

Over the past 50 years some rationing has taken place overtly, through waiting lists, local agreements to exclude procedures of limited effectiveness unless there are special clinical circumstances, and by controlling the introduction of expensive new technologies of marginal benefit. The majority of rationing, however, has occurred stealthily by dilution of existing services. Richard Smith in a *BMJ* editorial said '... choosing between resources spent on new drugs or on the number of nurses at night in geriatric wards or on facilities in the community for people with learning disabilities. Rationing in Britain works mostly by dilution rather than denial; it is politically so much easier particularly if you dilute services for the most marginal. Current policies which are biased toward the new rather than improving the infrastructure are increasing this as, for many managers it is now the only avenue of discretion.' This is the reality of the choices left to local managers when some choices are not available. It is the downside of moves to seek uniformity is some parts of the service only.

Problems are compounded, as there is real political reluctance to engage in an effective and public debate about these issues. There is an unwillingness to accept that if a community invests less in one thing it is because it invests more somewhere else, and to level up on whatever is the current political preference means levelling down on items that are not national priorities. The challenge for managers is that some of these local differences are, in fact, the services most beloved by local communities. There is always a political bias towards acute services and 'high tech' services and a lack of consistency in the assessment of benefit. Significant resources are being invested in services where the cost per QALY is very high at the expense of other services where the benefit is higher but the political gain is not so great. Which politician will make his or her name by denying someone with cancer potentially an average 2 more months of progression-free survival at a cost of £60,000 per QALY to allow significant extra investment in services for alcohol addiction? These decisions are, therefore, placed on local management who are asked to deliver comprehensive services, meet the needs of local communities and satisfy political imperatives around a large number of national priorities and targets. Health economics is rational but the decisions about investment are political. Not surprisingly, therefore, most local priorities are set covertly and without a scientific approach, as managers do their best to juggle expectations and reconcile the unreconcilable.

What do decision makers want from health economists?

So what would we need to make health economics more helpful to decision makers? First, more robust methodologies and informative data about benefits are needed to help in the identification of appropriate options and the full range of costs and benefits; this is not usually available. Research on new drugs often includes inappropriate clinical comparators coupled with poor assessment of cost per QALY. This is made more difficult by the poor information systems in the NHS, which do not track individual care other than in episodes of treatment and provide poor cost data. Implementation of the current NHS information strategy will begin to tackle this. Sadly however, the level of investment in information management and technology has been one of the local choices left to managers, and with the pressure on postcode prescribing it has been an area of inadequate investment, with managers unable to invest in the technology to help in the future because of the costs of new technologies today.

Second, most studies focus on the point of intervention (e.g. cost of thrombolytic treatment for stroke) rather than quantifying the whole systems change needed to make the drug or technology worthwhile. A drug may be clinically and cost effective in a trial but the implications and costs of introduction into mainstream clinical practice – for example early admission of all stroke patients to hospital needing new beds and the purchase of new scanners for every hospital – may make the whole programme non-cost effective. It is difficult to assess the entire benefits and costs of such a major change and partial analysis may give the wrong answer. This needs complex assessment across whole systems and care pathways rather than an isolated intervention alone.

Third, the major choices facing managers are between very different types of services with radically different objectives. The decision may be between investment in mental health services for people with severe and enduring mental health problems or in therapies for cancer, or in a new orthopaedic surgeon to allow more hip replacements. All these services need investment and how can one decide which group of patients will benefit most from new money? Programme marginal budgeting can help, but as yet this is inadequate because of the poor, non-patient centred data collected routinely by the NHS.

Fourth, we need to be more imaginative in engaging communities effectively in the assessment of values and in building these into local evaluations and priority setting. This needs open and honest discussion and consideration of the real local choices. In my health authority, for example, we already provide among the highest access rates to surgery and could also introduce every new and expensive drug but to do so will require reductions in other services. Rationally, we would ensure that we are efficient in all of expenditure and then look at the areas where we currently spend significantly more than other communities and reduce expenditure in these. We already know local providers are efficient when benchmarked nationally. We differ in only one significant way from the average health authority, in the very high number of community hospital beds provided locally – far more than any other health community nationally. These hospitals offer local services in a very rural community and I have no doubt that, in discussions with the population, they would be valued far more highly than new technologies. Handling this discussion requires more than the objectivity of rational assessment. This is a political debate, touching the emotions and innate conservatism of people, both clinicians and the public who often have radically opposed views. A long-term public debate is needed to change this and make people more aware of the true choices available. This needs a degree of political honesty, realism and courage.

Fifth, I would like clear and consistent advice from experts about what to stop as well as what to start coupled with well designed incentives to encourage and enable the release of resources from mainstream investment. Current mechanisms do not do this effectively and clinicians and trusts who make difficult but rational decisions to change investment can find themselves penalised financially as unit costs may rise.

Finally, I would like the difficult nature of managing this complexity at a local level to be recognised. Effective management requires flexibility to allow local diversity to be delivered within a broad national framework and manageable agenda. We need the space to achieve the best out of health economics.

Conclusion

In conclusion, local decision making is a political and historical issue rather than a rational one. Health economics can be a helpful tool when a simple question is defined. Most decisions, however, are much more complex and require a series of judgements to be made about a range of trade-offs. These include the balance between population and individual benefit; between central and local priorities; between the values of different stakeholders coupled with a need to protect the disadvantaged and respect diversity. We need to be happy as ugly ducklings rather than aspire to be swans. This is why we need high calibre managers to manage the complexity of the real world and find the 'both/and' not the 'either/or' and, as David Hunter says, 'to muddle through elegantly'.

CHAPTER 27

Realistic ways to understand economic decisions: the sociologist's perspective

Donald Light

Introduction

If economics is about the exchange and allocation of valued goods, then the discipline of economics has limited abilities to analyse or understand economic behaviour. For most, economic theory and research today is unable to take into account four major forces that shape economic behaviour: institutions, culture, history and power. Understanding the actual economic decisions in the practice of medicine through health economics puts one at a further disadvantage, because its methods and models derive predominantly from a microeconomic theory that is based on the decisions of rational individuals. Neither doctors nor patients may qualify for this role. Both, moreover, operate within a complex interactive system of the GP's practice or the consultant's firm and its evolving relationships with the PCT or hospital and with still larger institutional and political forces. In addition, most of the economic decisions in the NHS and in many other healthcare systems do not involve prices or money in ways analogous to buying a car, or a fleet of cars.

The basic economic model

In order to appreciate the dimensions of the problem here, let us summarise the basic model of microeconomics from a leading text:[1]

People act as individuals. Each individual has preferences regarding any given economic activity. She or he ranks them by priority and assigns them utilities, or quantitative measures of their ranking. Individuals then choose or act to maximise their utilities so that economic actions can be said to be complete (one's preferences are clearly ranked and complete) and transitive (one prefers in rank order).

Scarcity of everything – time, money, opportunities – is axiomatically ubiquitous, not in objective terms but because it is held that people are never satisfied, can never get enough – the 'theory of non-satiation'. This explains why everyone strives to maximise their utilities. Maximising one's utilities requires trade-offs that involve the opportunity costs of what can not do or buy as well as the benefits of what one can. In making trade-offs, individuals define their indifference curves, the distribution of trade-offs between two or more preferences that an individual is indifferent about. Thus one can plot and calculate individuals' utilities and indifference curves and opportunity costs in order to predict their economic behaviour.

In order to make this abstract model more concrete, the authors of this leading text use the example of Ivan, a Russian who earns 20 rubles a week. Ivan has two strong preferences, to drink vodka and eat cabbage. With his wages, he can buy up to 20 cabbages or up to 15 litres of vodka a week. Any cabbage he buys presents him with opportunity costs of less alcohol, and vice versa. The trade-offs between these two preferences form his 'indifference curve', which, of course, he wants to maximise. Looking at each end of the curve, Ivan is said to

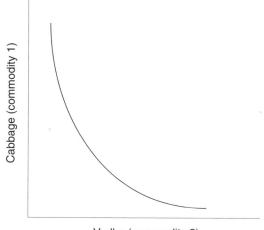

Figure 27.1: Ivan's indifference curve between cabbage and vodka. The curve shows the combinations of commodities that yield the same satisfaction or utility for Ivan.

be indifferent as to whether he spends his time eating nearly three cabbages a day and having no vodka, or having no cabbages and getting stone drunk on his home brew. Further, the model assumes that Ivan cannot get enough of either. Should his income rise to 30 rubles a week, he would eat more cabbages or drink himself to death, or (in combination) wash his cabbages down with his vodka – it does not matter which.*

Proper or formal markets and institutional actors are based on the axioms of this core theory of economic behaviour. Price theory is based on them. Most of the regulations and laws governing economic behaviour are based on these assumptions of how people behave. From a research perspective, the assumptions, principles and theory of economic behaviour can be tested as hypotheses. The research question is how accurately do they characterise people's economic behaviour? Do people have, as individuals, clear preferences, and do they rank them and employ them in making decisions and taking action? Each of the core assumptions of formal economic theory should be tested.

Limitations of the economic model

Applying microeconomics to healthcare is a relatively new undertaking. For decades, leading economists considered medicine to lack the basic prerequisites for price-competitive markets.[2–4] Clinical medicine is rife with uncertainties and too often contingent on diagnosis and response. Thus 'products' often cannot be defined, and property rights may be unclear. Physicians vary substantially in how they treat the same problem. Good market information is poor and highly asymmetrical. The absence of these requirements for beneficial competition can mean that competition is harmful to patients and society,[5] but it also means that economic models are limited in their ability to analyse actual economic decisions.

These serious misfits between the attributes of clinical medicine and the requirements for competition led Enthoven[6,7] to develop the theory of managed competition. To overcome these forms of market failure Enthoven emphasised competition between comprehensive healthcare plans and stipulated several requirements for a fair and beneficial market, such as universal health insurance

---

* The other chief example in Katz and Rosen is Elizabeth, who likes both tacos and hamburgers. As she is crunching her way through a dozen tacos, she is thinking of the opportunity costs of not having hamburgers; and when she's woofing down burgers, she's thinking about those tacos she could be having. Note the contraction between feeling deprived by the opportunity costs of what one cannot have and being 'indifferent' about whether Elizabeth eats 18 tacos and 2 hamburgers a week, or 18 hamburgers and 2 tacos.

or access, coverage of a common set of benefits, risk-adjusted contracts and good comparative information on quality, efficiency, and costs. He also held that healthcare markets had to be actively managed, because providers had proved so clever in manipulating or circumventing rules. Thus he called 'managed care' 'managed competition' rather than 'regulated competition'.

Managed competition appears to surmount the obstacles to effective markets in healthcare, and it is uncritically embraced as the model for making health-care services more efficient and responsive via competition. However, a careful analysis shows that the theory is seriously flawed, so that even if managed com-petition were implemented in its ideal form, it would not work as promised. First, managed competition leads to oligopolies forming in each market, and they would minimise the very competition the model aims to engender.[8,9] Second, managed competition assumes that providers cannot be trusted but managers can. Third, it also does not solve the problems of uncertainty or contingency or information asymmetry, but instead puts them inside its basic unit, the HMO, where Enthoven assumes that managers will resolve all these problems better than professionals did in the old market structure. As the inside literature on HMOs indicates, many of them remain unresolved or are resolved in disturbing ways.[10] For example, the broad overlapping networks of providers shared by plans that are supposedly competitive mean that:[11–13]

- the providers are in effect competing against themselves
- developing good clinical management tools and information is unlikely
- providers will be less interested in investing in a given plan's programme for clinical re-engineering
- plans can win contracts by paying providers less and limiting services more.

Managed competition also undermines public health and area-wide pro-grammes, although many small collaborations are celebrated.[14]

At a micro, empirical level, a leading American health economist, Tom Rice has summarised studies documenting several other practical problems.[15] First, the preferences of patients and employers are not fixed, but are affected by prior experience, current interactions and advertising. Rice believes this poses 'a very big problem' for researchers and competitors as well as for economic theory, as do problems posed by uncertainty and contingency. Second, consumers' choices do not necessarily reveal their preferences and may be poor judges of them. Third, Rice observes, consumers have poor market information, and fourth, when they are given it, studies find they sometimes ignore the most relevant data. Fifth, a majority of users are also unable to understand basic labels, instructions, and policies.[16] What, then, actually takes places in healthcare markets, especially when 'consumers' do not consume or buy, even though standard texts charac-terise them that way?[17]

A sociological approach to economic behaviour

Economic sociology is a burgeoning field in the United States and has resulted in numerous studies of complex economic behaviour. One might summarise its theory as follows:

People have relationships that shape their preferences and are shaped by them. The repertoire of preferences is largely provided by one's culture and location in society, as are the ways in which they are pursued. People's goals generally are to thrive and help others thrive within them, economically as well as in other ways. Thus, choice is based on reciprocity and on giving as well as gaining. 'Maximising one's utilities' would be regarded as greedy or selfish and be sanctioned by others in one's networks. Many economic choices have consequences for others, and people weigh these in making choices. That is, they weigh the harms or liabilities and benefits for others in deciding how to act. Thus relational choices are contingent and interdependent, not individualistic. No 'indifference curve' is possible, both because people are not indifferent about trade-offs between preferences and because various combinations of preferences for a given person have different benefits and consequences for oneself and others, and people are not indifferent to them.

Some goods and services are scarce but others are not. Some are plentiful, depending on tastes, circumstances, values and relationships. Most people can, and do, 'get enough' of many experiences, services and goods. Equilibrium consists of balanced reciprocal exchanges within a given network, community and culture. There is a goal, though not a principle, of satiation, including good relations and beneficial exchanges. Even if things are scarce, reciprocal exchanges enhance well being or satisfaction.

This theory of economic relationships and exchange is almost the obverse of the microeconomic model. It implies that the microeconomic model of behaviour is a theoretically constructed reality that has been used over time to construct contemporary markets. This implies that the means of pursuing preferences are socially constructed, even when they are constructed by neoclassical economists.

The historical context of economic transaction

For most of economic history nearly all economic transactions were informal, interpersonal and relational. In his historical essays, Polanyi[18] assembled evidence that most economic activity consisted of supporting households and governments, reciprocal or equivalency exchanges, gift exchanges, and contributions followed by redistributions. The first requirement for formal economic exchange is well defined and enforceable property rights within or between established political entities, and usually they did not exist. In his review of Polanyi's work, Douglass North, the Nobel Laureate in economics, agrees and points out that most historically oriented scholars agree as well, 'Polanyi maintains that reciprocity and redistribution were the dominant "transactional modes" in past societies and, increasingly, characterise economies in this century as well'.[19] There was no 'economy' aside from relations among households, institutions and governments. Exchanges were motivated by duty, kinship, friendship, religion and politics, not profit. Most exchanges took place without markets. Transaction costs and risks were very low, and trust very high. Some exchanges were formal in the sense of being institutionalised, ritualised or routinised. Many were informal. 'These substitutes for markets,' North wrote in modern corporate times, 'not only have dominated exchange in past societies, but do so today as well'.[19] He seemed to be thinking of informal and formal exchanges of time and services (and sometimes goods) inside firms, households, voluntary associations and governmental units, as well as exchanges between them. Five dimensions found in actual economic exchanges are value introjection, reciprocity, bounded solidarity, enforceable trust and trustworthiness.[20]

Economic behaviour in the real world

Economic behaviour begins with cognitive and cultural categories that get combined into scripts which actors routinely use in deciding what they value, buy or sell.[21] 'Cultural capital' and status competition influence economic scripts and decisions.[22] These scripts allow actors, whose capacity for rationality is bounded by their ability to filter, sort and apply what they know through 'selective attention'. The sociology of microeconomics, or actual market behaviour closely observed, looks more like a negotiated construction of a reality that the parties can live with, even if front-stage behaviour conforms to the scripts and symbols of market competition.[23] Institutionalised routines, once established, define paths which others follow, making future actions 'path dependent'. Most industries (and certainly healthcare) are 'oligopolies guarding carefully differentiated niches through strategies that aim to preserve rents by avoiding ruinous competition'.[24]

Conclusion

This chapter has demonstrated the deficiencies of applying a market model to resource decisions in healthcare and emphasised the importance of institutional setting, culture history and power. From a sociological perspective, key dimensions for analysing economic interactions in healthcare are:

- the relative frequency of transactions
- their relative complexity
- their relative specificity
- their relative size and risk
- their relative quality of information
- the degree of social relationship over time.

Each of these continua must be assessed in terms of each major party affected. Sociological dimensions of the relationships between parties in an economic transaction include:

- the degree of autonomy versus mutual obligations between them
- the degree of tightness or looseness in the network or organisation
- the size of the organisations or networks
- the structure of power relationships.

This approach is likely to provide a realistic analysis of economic decisions in clinical medicine and other realms of social life.

References

1   Katz ML and Rosen HS (1991) *Microeconomics*. Irwin, Homewood, IL.
2   Falk IS, Rorem CR and Ring MD (1933) *The Cost of Medical Care*. University of Chicago Press, Chicago.
3   Arrow K (1963) Uncertainty and the welfare economics of medical care. *Am Economic Rev.* **53**: 941–73.
4   Fox DM (1979) *Economists and Health Care: from reform to relativism*. Prodist, New York.
5   Light DW (1999) Good managed care needs universal health insurance. *Annals of Internal Medicine*. **130**: 686–9.
6   Enthoven A (1980) *Health Plan: the only practical solution to the soaring costs of medical care*. Addison-Wesley, Reading, MA.
7   Enthoven A (1988) *Theory and Practice of Managed Competition in Health Care Finance*. North-Holland, Amsterdam.
8   Light DW (1995) *Homo economicus*: escaping the traps of managed competition. *Eur J Public Health*. **5**: 145–54.
9   Sullivan K (1995) *Strangled Competition: a critique of Minnesota's experiment with managed competition*. COACT Educational Foundation, St Paul.
10 Anon (1998) *Managed Care Challenges: health system change brief*. Center for Studying Health System Change, Washington DC.

11   Eddy DM (1998) Performance measurement: problems and solutions, *Health Affairs.* **17(4):** 7–25.

12   Ginsberg P (1998) *A Perspective on Health System Change in 1997.* Center for Studying Health System Change, Annual Report. Washington DC, 1–9.

13   Sullivan K (1997) *Strangled Competition II: the quality of care under managed competition.* COACT Educational Foundation, St Paul.

14   Lasker RD (1997) *Medicine & Public Health: the power of collaboration.* Academy of Medicine, New York.

15   Rice T (1998) *The Economics of Health Reconsidered.* Health Administration Press, Chicago.

16   American Medical Association (1999) Health literacy: report of the Council on Scientific Affairs. *JAMA.* **281:** 552–7.

17   Folland S, Goodman AC and Stano M (1997) *The Economics of Health and Health Care.* Prentice-Hall, Upper Saddle River, NJ.

18   Polanyi K (1944) *The Great Transformation.* Reinhart, New York.

19   North DC (1977) Markets and other allocation systems in history: the challenge of Karl Polanyi. *J Eur Economic History.* **6:** 703–16.

20   Portes A and Sesenbrenner J (1993) Embeddedness and immigration: notes on the social determinants of economic action. *Am J Socio.* **98:** 1320–50.

21   Dimaggio P (1997) Culture and cognition. *Ann Rev Socio.* **24:** 263–87.

22   Portes A (1998) Social capital: its origins and applications in modern sociology. *Ann Rev Socio.* **24:** 1–24.

23   Hughes D, Griffiths L and McHale JV (1997) Do quasi-markets evolve? Institutional analysis and the NHS. *Cambridge J Economics.* **21:** 259–76.

24   DiMaggio P (1998) The new institutionalism: avenues of collaboration. *J Institutional Theoretical Economics.* **154:** 696–705.

CHAPTER 28

Towards a behavioural health economics: the psychologist's perspective

Paul Webley

Introduction

A search through the electronic bibliographies reveals surprisingly few articles that deal with both health economics and psychology. Indeed, health economics seems more dominated by a broadly neoclassical approach (the market as the most efficient way to allocate resources within which individuals act rationally to maximise their utility) than mainstream economics itself, where there has been a steady stream of work heavily influenced by psychology (sometimes called 'behavioural economics')[1] and where Nobel laureates are happy to make use of psychological concepts such as identity.[2] Does this neglect of psychology matter? I think it does.

Economics does not just describe reality – it helps legitimise a particular view of reality (which makes its prescriptive use problematic.) This chapter considers the neglect of psychology by health economics and suggests that marrying the top-down approach of economics with the bottom-up approach of psychologists will lead to a more applicable and usable discipline.

Critique of health economics from a psychological perspective

Although there are some honourable exceptions,[3] what is striking to an outsider is that those working in health economics seem largely to take the standard economic assumptions for granted. Individuals are assumed to maximise their well being (utility), to have stable preferences and to take decisions in a rational manner. So if Fred prefers being seen by Dr Ash (kind, out-of-date) to being seen by Dr Beagle (curt but efficient), and prefers Dr Beagle to Dr Clarendon (courteous, up-to-date), he would prefer Dr Ash to Dr Clarendon (this is the axiom – note the terminology – of transitivity). Similarly, institutions are assumed to operate efficiently (to maximise profit if in private hands). The approach is top-down (from theoretical assumptions or axioms down to behaviour), analytical, rigorous and individualistic; units – whether individuals or institutions – are assumed always to being striving to selfishly maximise their utility.

Now, it is reasonably easy to show that these assumptions are sometimes wrong. If people were presented with choices between pairs of hypothetical general practitioners, for example, it is certain that not all the choices would be transitive, nor would they all be consistent from one week to the next (from previous studies we'd expect about 20% of choices to change each week). The usual response of economists to such findings is to concede that while it is true that on the individual level the axioms fail, this is irrelevant. What matters is whether detailed economic predictions or estimates are correct on average. This pragmatic defence of rationality has some force, but there are at least two areas relevant to health where it is certainly unconvincing. Let's look at each in turn.

Stable preferences in changing contexts

The first is the assumption of stable preferences. The value of anything (a year of good health or judgements of the quality of an individual's life, for instance) is assumed to be independent of how choices are presented or the context. However, actually goods and services tend to have one value to an individual in one context and a quite different value in another. This means that valuation studies (e.g. of the benefits to society of particular health policies) may well give distorted results.

The best known example of such context dependence is the asymmetric evaluation of gains and losses, which was first identified by Kahneman and Tversky,[4] and has subsequently been shown to hold in a wide variety of situations. Put simply, people are much more concerned about losses than they are about gains. We can see this memorably in the so-called endowment effect. If you split people into two groups, and give each member of one group a mug worth about 5 euros (and the other half nothing), those 'endowed' with a mug will typically value the mug at around 7 euros, whereas those without will value it at around $3\frac{1}{2}$ euros. Why? After all, a mug is a mug is a mug. One explanation is that those people given a mug very quickly incorporate it in their possessions (it becomes 'their' mug). To leave without a mug is a loss, and it is a loss for which one must

---

Box 28.1:   Two scenarios that have the same outcome

If programme A is adopted, 200 people will be saved.
If programme B is adopted there is a 1/3 probability that 600 people will be saved and a 2/3 probability that no people will be saved.

OR

If programme C is adopted, 400 people will die.
If programme D is adopted there is a 1/3 probability that nobody will die and a 2/3 probability that 600 people will die.

---

be compensated. Whereas the reference point for those who never had one is different; acquiring the mug is a gain, and gains are valued less than losses.

Reference points turn out to be crucial in a wide range of judgements. In the mug example, people really did have different reference points (some were lucky enough to have been given one). However, we can show another important gain–loss effect if the situation is framed in different ways. The classic example comes from Tversky and Kahneman again.[5] Participants were presented with various hypothetical problems. In one of these, people had to imagine that a country was threatened with a disease that was expected to kill 600 people. They then had to make a choice between two alternative interventions. These two alternatives were described in two different ways shown in Box 28.1.

These are obviously the same choices described in different ways (with 600 people at risk 200 people saved is the same as 400 people dying). However, if people were given the first version 72% opted for programme A, whereas if they were given the second version 78% went for programme D. What this shows is a general tendency for people to be risk-averse for gains and risk-seeking for losses – put another way, sure gains are popular whereas sure losses are unpopular.

One possible response to this kind of study is to claim that framing and other context effects are only important when the situation is hypothetical. This is not the case – the differing effects of gains and losses can also be seen, for example, in the very real world of tax paying. Another response is to claim that these effects are trivial, only found in the psychology laboratory and that with experience they will disappear. Again, this is not true. Perhaps the most compelling demonstration of this is a recent study by Harbaugh *et al.*[6] who show that children of all ages are just as susceptible to the endowment effect as adults – years of experience seem to make no difference at all. Health economists, therefore, have to take this kind of evidence seriously and develop theories and models that take context effects into account. They should also consider using the minimum sum people would accept (WTA) to give up something rather than using willingness to pay (WTP) in valuing the benefits of healthcare programmes, as the value as an avoided loss is best measured using WTA.

Taking time into account

The second area is the economic psychology of time. The standard approach in health economics when dealing with future events is to assume that individuals 'discount' the future. That is, they would rather have things (goods, services) in the present than in the future (they might die, something else might go wrong) – so £1000 in a year's time is 'discounted' and is worth say £900 now. To assess the present value of alternative programmes, therefore, one discounts depending on when the benefits occur. That is fair enough (although it is worth noting that people typically show very high subjective discount rates indeed – they would very much rather have things now!). For an individual's choices to be consistent over time, the discount rate has to be constant. The evidence, however, suggests that people's choices over time are anything but consistent. So while someone might prefer £10 now to £20 in 4 months time, they may well nonetheless prefer £20 in 16 months time to £10 in a year's time. This makes good intuitive sense and has also been demonstrated in the health area by Van der Pol and Cairns.[7] They have shown a similar effect by asking people to imagine being ill at some point in the future and offering the opportunity for this period of ill health to be delayed as a result of treatment. Respondents had to identify the maximum number of days of future ill health for which it would still be worth receiving the treatment. The further in the future the illness was anticipated to start, the lower the discount rate.

What this very general tendency implies is that, in financial matters, people save less (e.g. for their pension) than their future selves would like and, in health matters, that they behave in ways (e.g. overeat) that have deleterious long-term consequences. Finding strategies to overcome this problem is important both for individuals and society.[8]

I've only briefly discussed two areas relevant to health where the failure of the standard economic model seems to have particularly serious repercussions – there are, of course, lots of others (for a short general introduction to the field of economic psychology see Webley et al.[9]). The important take-away message is that aspects of the standard model are seriously flawed and could be improved if a more bottom-up approach, which takes into account how people really think and act, was used.

A possible defence to the line of argument that I have put forward here is that while the assumptions underpinning health economics may not make up a good descriptive model of the way people act and think, they do offer a prescriptive or normative standard. In other words, while individuals may be irrational, use rules of thumb (rather than assessing alternative courses of actions exhaustively), have unstable preferences and so on, those people responsible for making policy recommendations must not be. There are three problems with this. First, in order to carry out cost benefit analyses, one needs measures of the costs and benefits involved and some of these have to be derived from individuals. Therefore, we have to understand how individuals make their judgements, and how they think about their health and healthcare options. Second, GPs, service managers and the like, who have to implement policy, are human too; we need to understand how they might make use of the economic information that is provided to them. Third, current economics, based as it is on self-interest and rationality is itself part of the problem.

This probably sounds overstated. Let us pause to consider. People are selfish but they also have moral concerns, and values matter. They are individuals but aren't just individuals; they are better thought of as members of a culture that creates and sustains different value systems. From this perspective (essentially that put forward in Etzioni's *The Moral Dimension*[10]), standard economics is not describing reality but is contributing to legitimising a particular – amoral – approach to life. This suggests that we should be very careful before using the results of economic analyses as normative or prescriptive.

Moving forward: the behavioural agenda in health economics

It is always easier to be critical than to be constructive. Given my comments above, is there a way forward for health economics? Is it possible to marry a top-down approach (with its rigour, clarity and analytical power) with a bottom-up approach (with an emphasis on empirical studies of the messiness of the real world)? Can we put communitarian values and morals back into health economics?

I think it is fair to say that many economists worry about losing analytical power – they know that many of their assumptions are wrong, but are certain that 'naïve empiricism' will get them nowhere and concerned about the mathematical intractability of alternative approaches to modelling the world. However, there are things that can be done. Perhaps most important is the development of new theories which capture important psychological processes. These need to combine the rigour and mathematical elegance of the best economic models with the insights of economic psychologists and other social scientists. They will treat people not as isolated units but as members of families, communities and organisations. Decision making is rarely truly individual; even apparently private decisions (such as contraceptive use) are heavily influenced by social norms and what is fashionable (a very social concept). As well as new theories, health economists also need to make much more extensive use of qualitative methods, as these give a greater insight into the social and psychological processes involved in health decision making (of individuals, health practitioners and managers). This does not mean abandoning quantitative methods, which are vital, but supplementing them with alternative approaches that provide new insights.[11]

Health economists also need to keep on eye on work by economic psychologists, who are just beginning to take an interest in health matters.[12] This approach is non-normative, empirical and has the individual subjective experience of health as its starting point. It puts the individual at the heart of the research programme and treats them as a consumer of goods and services. It is early days yet, but so far this approach has identified different behavioural styles of healthcare consumers, perceptions of the quality of service provided by GPs and insight into the subjective experience of health and illness.

I have no easy blueprint for success (I wish I did). But I am certain that focusing on real individuals, with all their complexities and apparent inconsistencies will help health economics get into practice.

References

1   Rabin M (1998) Psychology and economics. *J Economic Literature.* **36(1):** 11–46.
2   Akerlof GA and Kranton RE (2000) Economics and identity. *Quarterly J Economics.* **115(3):** 715–53.
3   Shiell A, Seymour J, Hawe P and Cameron S (2000) Are preferences over health states complete? *Health Economics.* **9(1):** 47–55.
4   Kahneman D and Tversky A (1979) Prospect theory: an analysis of decision under risk. *Econometrica.* **47:** 263–91.
5   Tversky A and Kahneman D (1981) The framing of decisions and the psychology of choice. *Science.* **211:** 453–8.
6   Harbaugh WT, Krause K and Vesterlund L (2001) Are adults better behaved than children? Age, experience, and the endowment effect. *Economics Letters.* **70(2):** 175–81.
7   Van der Pol M and Cairns J (In press) A comparison of the discounted utility model and hyperbolic discounting models in the case of social and private intertemporal preferences for health. *J Economic Behav Organization.*
8   Ainslie G (1992) *Picoeconomics.* Cambridge University Press, Cambridge.
9   Webley P, Burgoyne CB, Lea SEG and Young BM (2001) *The Economic Psychology of Everyday Life.* Psychology Press, Hove.
10 Etzioni A (1988) *The Moral Dimension: towards a new economics.* Free Press, New York.
11 Coast J (1999) The appropriate uses of qualitative methods in health economics. *Health Economics.* **8(4):** 345–53.
12 Pepermans R, Groenland E, Bloem S and Staipers J (2001) Towards a consumer based healthcare behaviour model: a behavioural process approach. In: AJ Scott (ed) *Environment and Wellbeing: proceedings of the 26th Annual Colloquium of IAREP.* University of Bath, Bath, 225–8.

CHAPTER 29

Thinking it through: a philosophical perspective

Martyn Evans

The economist's challenge

One of the most valuable things the health economist does for us is to challenge us. Why should we not attempt to obtain the most good for a given expenditure, or spend least in order to achieve a given good? Is this not the most responsible approach to dispensing funds which (in the NHS) may be public property, all-too-scarce, and held in stewardship for the relief of suffering and disability? What could be more moral than trying to make these funds work hardest for us?

I think we could accept the moral truth underlying these questions; and if we could accept it then it seems that we therefore should. The question then is whether the methods and assumptions of the health economist offer us the best practical means to getting the result we want, and connectedly whether they do so without incurring a different sort of cost, and one that we might not want to pay.

I am going to focus on this latter point, the point about the kinds of costs which we might find ourselves facing – but might not wish to face. They won't in themselves be economic costs. They won't even, I suspect, be the kind of costs the economist can actually describe or say much about. Economists usually (and wisely) try to confine themselves to pointing out the different kinds of 'goods' that compete for our attention and our resources. This competing can be described in terms of how committing ourselves to one 'good' results in losing the opportunity to acquire any of the others. 'Cost' is, for the economist, 'opportunity cost'. However, not all goods can be distinguished or costed in economic terms, as some goods can neither be obtained nor given up in strict competition with one another.

'Beyond compare'?

Think, for example, of curiosity, the tang of sea air, the gentle patina of mellow red bricks, a kindly word after (or indeed before) a vexing day at the office, the blazing exultation of a try scored in rugby, parental pride or a sunset. Each of these could, no doubt, be considered as being in competition with some other 'good' of the same or a similar kind, or something obtained with a comparable kind of effort. So the tang of sea air might in some rather stretched sense 'compete' with the musk of crushed heather on the moors, insofar as you could drive for, say, an hour from home in either of two opposite directions, park your car, and breathe a deep draught of one of these two scented delights – but not both simultaneously nor, perhaps, in the same half-day away from the office. Mellow red bricks might 'compete' for your favours with wooden clap-board facings if you were planning your dream home in Kent. The (for me) peerless excitement of a well-run try in rugby union might perhaps 'compete' with some other sporting thrill, such as the long-resisted overtaking manoeuvre in a long-distance track race, if you could watch only one such event in an afternoon. But these comparisons rely on putting my different examples in appropriate categories, and matching them against other examples within those same categories. Even here, the results are rather strained. They become ludicrous when trying to compare the examples from different categories.

Moreover some of the examples – I'm thinking particularly of curiosity itself, or of parental pride – defy being put into categories at all. What other kind of thing is there that is 'like' curiosity, or parental pride? Hence, what else could possibly claim the same part of our ambition or satisfaction as parental pride? What else could possibly take the place of curiosity? Even to frame the question sounds faintly unhinged.

There is a whole range of what I would like to call 'intangible' goods of this sort. And curiously, given their other obvious limitations, prime ministers are as adept at naming these more intangible goods as they are clumsy in trying to manufacture them. Mrs Margaret Thatcher pointed to a range of goods previously and perhaps more authoritatively identified by Saint Francis of Assisi, including the systematic replacement of injury by pardon, doubt by faith, despair by hope, darkness by light and sadness by joy. For his part Mr John Major aspired to a nation which was 'at ease with itself'. Mr Tony Blair proclaimed the values of justice and progress and community, together with the courage necessary to take practical measures in pursuit of noble causes. There is of course nothing wrong with wanting these things, and nothing wrong with naming them. But there are some things you cannot do with them.

Troubles with counting and dividing

You can't count them, for instance. Nor can you divide them up. I do not know who was the wag who coined the term 'milli-Helen' for that degree of facial beauty 'just sufficient to launch one ship'. Facial – or any other kind of – beauty is indivisible. That doesn't mean that some faces are not more beautiful than some others; of course they are. But not all differences are differences in measurable quantity. And the fact that you can have more of something than someone else does not mean that it makes the slightest sense to say quantifiably how much of it you have, or how much of it they have.

Beauty is only one example. Well being seems to me to be another. So do fulfilment, personal satisfaction, self-actualisation, dignity, curiosity and individuality. We could reasonably desire all of these things, if only because they are by definition desirable – though we could not all reasonably expect to get them all. Perhaps sometimes the pursuit of one of them (for instance, well being, or curiosity) happens at the expense of another of them (for instance, individuality, or dignity). I notice that I've fallen into using a very economic-sounding word, namely 'expense', in this last sentence. While it seems obvious to me that, say, curiosity could lead me into some very undignified situations, I certainly didn't want to appear to suggest an economic transaction between curiosity and dignity.

In particular, I didn't want to suggest that the economic notion of 'opportunity cost' covers the balance between these two intangible goods. ('trade-off', the image that comes immediately to mind, shows in itself perhaps how successful the economic or commercial model has been in coming to dominate so many of our rather unthinking metaphors.) The reason that 'opportunity cost' is inadequate here is that it seems to rely on there being some notion of convertibility between the opportunities. Otherwise, how could they be regarded as in competition? We must assume that energy or resources devoted to one could have been devoted to another. This at least is a minimal form of convertibility – the convertibility of consumption of effort or resource, and moreover of consumption of comparable or even equivalent resource. But that requires that the goods which are the subject of the opportunities be to some degree measurable or quantified. The tang of the sea was 'one hour's drive' worth of effort, as was the musk of the heather-clad moors. But this is a poor equivalence. I might have been prepared to drive farther for the one than for the other; yet I guess I'd be completely at a loss to say how much farther I'd have driven before the effort seemed no longer worthwhile.

The economist's approach, perfectly naturally and reasonably, relies on our concentrating on things which can be measured, quantified. Just like evidence-based medicine, it directs our energies to outcomes which can be numerically demonstrated, hence which can somehow be converted into numbers in the first place. So things which cannot be converted into numbers are to say the least inconvenient, a distraction, and best set aside. We should (on this picture) devote our energies to things which can be measured and quantified, so that we can show the return on our investment. Thus the intangibles will, by default, systematically be at best neglected and at worst suppressed.

Other sorts of cost

It is the non-economic cost of having and then losing 'goods' of this more elusive kind that concern me as a philosopher. It is hard to talk about the costs of losing them without sounding either pompous or discouraging. At least I ought to make it clear that I certainly don't complain at economists for not calculating them; generally speaking, they wisely do not try.

Now when we find that our health is compromised, and we seek medical advice and treatment, we often find that striving to restore our normal state of health does involve losing some of these other intangible goods, to some extent. But then how do we decide whether these costs are ultimately worth paying? Clearly, we cannot be surprised that there are costs of this kind, any more than we could be surprised at having to acknowledge the persistence of intangible things that make life rich and interesting.

Which of these intangible costs are then involved, indeed embedded, in the health economist's otherwise compelling enterprise? For me, they principally concern what happens when we standardise the way we look at and describe individual patients, for the purposes of working out how much they could potentially benefit from receiving a certain treatment, or of working out how much they actually have benefited. The trouble is, I believe, that this is very difficult in practical terms, and indeed neglectful of the individuality and richness of patients' lives. Standardising people means downgrading or, indeed, actually suppressing what makes them different as individuals.

In that sense it is also rather objectionable, even in the moral sense of the word 'objectionable'. We have to turn people into units of healthcare consumption, or into standardised organisms with sets of nominal functional ranges. As units of consumption they become items on the debit side of the healthcare balance sheet, and as such a kind of threat to the fiscal dimension of the nation's health. Simply obtaining 'the most healthcare per pound spent' is not in itself threatened by the corresponding consumption of that healthcare. Indeed, economists will tell us that without consumption (represented on the 'demand side' of any economic arrangement) transactions will soon stop. Healthcare actually needs the sick, in this sense – it actually needs them to use up what the NHS has to offer. But what we think constitutes 'the most healthcare per pound spent' now comes into the equation.

Can people be standardised?

From the point of view of economics in isolation, it probably doesn't matter if all the consumption is accounted for by a very few, very sick, individuals – if as a result of that consumption they get very much better, and constitute a demonstrably very large return on our investment. The unit of return, in this sense, is a measure of radical and dramatic recovery. A big return is therefore any 'big' recovery, from deep morbidity or pathology, without much concern for who the patients are or how many of them there are. An individual with a heavy consumption of healthcare is not a problem in this picture – she or he is simply a convenient locus for showing the return on our money.

But this is hardly likely to appeal to us as a complete picture of what we want the NHS to do. Our ideas about producing very large amounts of healthcare are more likely to consist in somehow successfully treating very large numbers of people. The unit of return now is simply one patient, or more sophisticatedly perhaps one discrete pathology tied to an identifiable and discrete patient. A big return means treating as many people, or as many different pathologies, as possible. In that context, someone who incurs a heavy individual consumption of healthcare is a kind of threat. One very sick, very resource-hungry person stands in the way of a 'big return' measured in terms of the several other people who could have been treated for that same expenditure.

I am going to assume that the unattractiveness of thinking about people in this way is obvious enough and would be acknowledged by most readers of this book. It seems unkind to think of someone with very great need as being automatically a problem for a hypothetical group of other people, each having individually much smaller needs. It seems unkind to try to equate people in this way. The problem for me is that this way of thinking is also the natural result of trying to 'equate' people at all, in the sense of standardising them for the purposes of measuring the amounts by which they are needy, or the amounts by which they can benefit. We feel that in order to take need seriously, we want to think of someone's individual need in their context (what the need means for them), and not in the context of a lot of other needs which we can easily find, in great if not overwhelming numbers.

The centrality of experience

So what does the patient's need mean for them? The answer to this is to be found in their experience of their health state, illness or disability, and the healthcare interventions intended to help them. I think the patient's experiences are clinically central in ways which intensify the importance of involvement, of being interested, and of caring about what one does, in the pursuit of quality in healthcare. This is something which it will be difficult to measure, and hence difficult to apportion – fairly or unfairly.

First, the primary activity of healthcare concerns experiences as such – that is, the experiences of suffering (principally bodily suffering) and its relief. If a condition doesn't involve suffering or incapacity, or if it isn't going to lead to suffering or incapacity in the future, then the key reason for seeking or providing medical help is missing. And both suffering and incapacity are essentially experiences. How does the economist convincingly measure the intensity and range of these experiences in the only sense that really matters – the subjective sense, the lived, felt, experience of the patient? If this can't be done (and it seems surpassingly difficult) then a central ingredient of economic assessment seems to be missing.

Second, a meaningful specification of a healthcare outcome must typically include the patient's experience of the process of healthcare interventions. Even if we could sometimes detach outcome from process – even if, say, a functionally satisfactory hernia repair stayed longer in the memory than the brusque or uninvolved or uninterested attitude of over-stretched contract nurses or junior doctors covering for sick colleagues or superiors – the patient's experiences of the clinical encounters still matter in their own right. 'Value for money' in healthcare terms seems a hollow notion if it fails to reflect the way in which the processes are delivered, which is to say, experienced by the patient. Do 'customer satisfaction' questionnaires give any real insight into this on an individual level?

My point is to acknowledge how important it is to attempt such measurement, but also and more significantly to point to the breadth of the range of data that are needed, including what we could call experiential data about how patients experience their suffering and incapacity, their contact with the health service, and their wider social and domestic stories. But the trouble is (or so it seems to me) that these experiential data are highly resistant to being captured in any kind of scale. We may produce visual analogue scales, and we may calibrate or ratify or validate or 'triangulate' these by repeated use with large numbers of patients. When we have done this to our satisfaction, can we then claim that a point one-third of the way along the scale represents precisely, or even remotely, half as much of the phenomenon in question as compared to a 'reading' two-thirds of the way along the same scale? I doubt it. Partly I doubt it because I am not convinced that averaging out very many subjective answers gives you an 'objective' answer in its place. Partly I doubt it because the reality of an experience is a matter of the moment of having it, and the memory of one earlier experience seems at an inherent disadvantage compared to the impact of now actually having a new experience. But mainly I doubt it because even for a single person to say, sincerely and after careful reflection, that one pain is twice as intense as another, or that one cannula was inserted only half as gently as the previous one, or that the décor and regimen in one elderly care unit is twice as caring, life-affirming or individually sensitive as in a previous unit, may be an imaginative and picturesque way of saying 'more' or 'less' but is – frankly speaking – absurd if taken literally in the quantitative sense which the economist seeks.

I appreciate that in order to say that one experience is better than another we seem to feel the need to say by how much it was better, in some common coin, in amounts of some units or other. But goodness, and betterness – quality in general – just doesn't seem to come in units. Nor do most of the other things we might pick out as qualities, be they positive or negative. There are no really convincing units, so far as I can see, of relief, restfulness, tranquillity, irritation, painfulness, miserableness, depression, tightness, relaxedness, politeness, rudeness, or of any of the other qualities that we might think important in evaluating the healthcare experience. We would do better to find ways of capturing experiences in words rather than in numbers.

For instance, if someone felt that her reduced joint mobility was a price worth paying, for the less severe nausea caused by the alternative anti-inflammatory drug, that would be an important experiential datum. The datum is irreducibly personal, not easily generalised, and not quantifiable; it has to be described in words.

Conclusion

None of these restrictions makes the datum less valuable – indeed, they show the special way in which it is valuable. But that special way is, I think, one which resists the economist's preferred use of it. It resists being fed into an accumulated sum of equal or comparable preferences on the part of other people, because there seems no intelligible way of showing that other preferences are equal or comparable to it. 'Sums' of such preferences are, in consequence, a poor basis for working out the fairest or most effective distribution of our healthcare resources.

The economist is right to challenge us to do 'the most good' with the limited means available to us. If we could do it, and know when we'd done it, the challenge would be morally compelling. Readers of this book must decide for themselves whether, or how far, healthcare outcomes can be quantified in this way. For the reasons given here, I personally remain sceptical.

CHAPTER 30

Health economics and insights from complexity theory

David Kernick

'Those who take for their standard anyone but nature weary themselves in vain.'

Leonardo de Vinci

Introduction

Models help us to see pattern in the world around us. We create reality around 'bundles of related assumptions', conceptual lenses through which we view the world. In this chapter, we explore the emerging science of complex adaptive systems that offers a complementary perspective on organisations and is already finding an application within healthcare.

Underpinned by the mathematical analyses of chaos theory, the focus moves to the non-linear configuration of relationships among a system's components and an understanding of what creates patterns of order and behaviour among them. The important features are connectivity, diversity, feedback and the existence of self-ordering rules that give systems the capacity to emerge to new patterns of order. Complexity theory offers us a more relevant model with which to view the real world where we operate under the constraints of limited time, knowledge and processing power, and where the bulk of our activity is to establish and modify relationships through time rather than seeking an endless series of goals each of which disappear on attainment. It is an approach that resonates with the experience of practitioners and healthcare managers and is beginning to make an impact on a broad range of disciplines. This chapter briefly describes some of these complexity insights and their challenge to health economics.

The development of modern science and the dominance of linearity

The period of the enlightenment that began in the late eighteenth century, was based on the confident assumption that the application of reason would expand knowledge and purge the residues of religion and mysticism. Human progress was to be achieved by a programme that extended scientific knowledge and technical control to all aspects of society. The predominant model for modern science was to be the machine, underpinned by three main assumptions.

- Reductionism – a system can be understood by breaking it down and understanding its component parts. The behaviour of the system can be inferred from the sum of its parts.
- Linearity – there is a simple and proportional relationship between inputs (cause) and outputs (effect) for any part of the machine.
- Determinism – a knowledge of the component parts will predict the future.

In this model of a 'clockwork universe', an independent observer can stand outside the system and engineer it towards defined objectives (Box 30.1). Complicated systems need complicated rules and when these do not yield the required results, even more rules must be created.

Health economics sits within the modernist view of the world. Thus, society is composed of individuals who act in a predictable fashion to maximise their utility, and the welfare of society is the sum of the utilities of these autonomous individuals. There is always a simple relationship between inputs and outputs at any system level. Context, non-equilibrium and interrelationships are not accommodated within the model. Approximations and statistical manipulations are used to adjust for discrepancies while predictive limitations are viewed as data or processing inadequacies, omissions, bias or randomness.

Box 30.1: Elements of the 'modern' approach to problems in healthcare

- *Reductionist* – systems can be understood by breaking them down into their component parts.
- *Linear* – there is a simple relationship between inputs and outputs. Small inputs have small effects, large inputs have large effects.
- *Deterministic* – the future of a system can be predicted with certainty.
- *Rational/analytical* – problems can be formulated as the making of a rational choice between alternative means of achieving a known end.
- *Impartiality* – an observer can stand outside the system without being influenced by it and engineer it towards defined objectives.

The rise of non-linearity – chaos theory and the study of complex adaptive systems

]Although the linear model of modern science has had many spectacular successes, when applied to health service organisation and delivery, there does seem to be some cause for concern. For example, research seems to have little direct influence on health service policy;[1] health economists continue to develop technical solutions that find little impact at grassroots level;[2] rational priority setting remains elusive;[3] managers demonstrate a predilection for process rather than outcome indicators;[4] and practitioners are reluctant to follow evidence-based guidelines.[5] Why should this be?

All systems are linear when close to equilibrium. However, social systems are constantly changing and remain far from equilibrium limiting analysis within a linear framework. Converging from a number of disciplines, complexity theory recognises that many systems comprise of networks of elements interacting constantly to give rise to behaviour that is not predictable and which cannot be understood by breaking down the system into its component parts. The reason for this unpredictable behaviour is the presence of positive and negative feedback loops in the system which are acting recursively (repetitively and feeding back on themselves) which give rise to non-linear features as summarised in Box 30.2.

The quantitative analysis of non-linear systems is known as chaos theory. (A different meaning from its lay interpretation.) This science has opened up new analytical possibilities in physics and physiology ranging from the description of weather systems to cardiac function. Here, the reiterative feedback formulas that give rise to non-linearity remain constant and can be analysed mathematically. However, in social systems, the algorithms or 'mental models' that form the basis of individual interaction continually change and evolve as we learn. This put

---

Box 30.2: Characteristics of non-linear interactions

- They are unpredictable.
- Small changes can have large system effects.
- Large effects can lead to small system changes.
- Non-linear systems are sensitive to initial conditions – the history of the system is important.
- Non-linear systems cannot be understood by reduction into their component parts – the whole is different from the sum of the parts.

limits on formal quantitative analysis. Complexity can be seen as the qualitative study of non-linearity drawing upon the metaphors that chaos theory offers.

Fundamentals of complexity

In this section, we look at some of the principles of complexity and how they might offer us some new descriptive and prescriptive insights.

Complex systems

A complex system is a system of individual agents, who have the freedom to act in ways that are not always predictable, and whose actions are interconnected such that one agent's actions changes the context for other agents. The interaction between agents is invariably non-linear due to the existence of recursive feedback loops. Examples of complex systems include the immune system, the brain, a patient–doctor consultation, a hospital, or an entire health system. Complex systems have a number of unique features:[6]

- They consist of a large number of elements that interact dynamically by exchanging energy or information. The effects of these interactions are propagated throughout the system.
- They have many direct and indirect feedback loops.
- They exchange energy or information with their environment and operate at conditions far from equilibrium.
- They have memory, not located at a specific place, but distributed throughout the system and thus have a history.
- They have emergent properties – behaviour of the systems is determined by the nature of the interactions, not by what is contained within the components. As the interactions are rich, dynamic, and non-linear, the behaviour of the system as a whole cannot be predicted from an inspection of its components.
- They are adaptive – they can organise internal structure without the intervention of an external agent.

Arising from these features are a number of important concepts.

Mental models

Agents operate according to their own internal rules or mental models – rules for how they respond to the environment. As agents can both change and share their internal rules, complex systems can learn and adapt over time. Complexity is the result of the rich non-linear interaction of agents in response to the information each of them is presented with. An important insight is that the internal rules of agents and their subsequent actions may not predominately be influenced by an organisation's legitimate systems of hierarchy, rules and communication patterns but by the 'shadow organisation' that lies behind the scenes (e.g. hallway conversations).[7]

Complex systems are dependent on their history

As non-linear systems are dependent on initial conditions, the history of a system will be critical to an understanding of it and its development. For example, it would be inadvisable to consider the current developments in primary care in the NHS without an understanding of their historical context.

Information gets disseminated across a whole system

Although agents interact strongly with elements closest to them, information about such events may be communicated across the whole system. Due to non-linear characteristics, small changes in one area can occasionally have large effects across the whole system. This has been called the 'butterfly effect'. (A butterfly in New York can flap its wings and cause a hurricane in Tokyo.) For example, the riding accident of the actor Christopher Reeves had a large but probably inappropriate impact on the redistribution of research funding into spinal injuries in the United States.[8] Conversely, large influences may only have a negligible impact. *The Health of the Nation* initiative was a major strategic UK government initiative designed to influence the health of the public but had little impact on the targets it sought to influence.[9]

Because of this distributed non-linearity, detailed planning and prediction is never possible. This insight has been interpreted as 'good enough vision'. For example, rather than spend time on detailed planning and striving to calculate a solution by the continuous addition of rules, planners should be content with setting minimum specifications and establishing boundaries and letting the system settle into a condition that satisfies the constraints placed on it.

Complex systems are unpredictable but have emergent properties

Although unpredictable, the behaviour of complex systems evolves from the interaction of agents at a local level, without external direction or the presence of internal control. This property is known as emergence and gives systems the flexibility to adapt and self-organise in response to external challenge. Emergence is a pattern of system behaviour that could not have been predicted by an analysis of the component parts of that system. A balance of cooperation and competition drives change in such a way as to maintain system stability. A self-organising system will attempt to balance itself at a point known as self-organised criticality where it is able to adapt with the least amount of effort. The system will seek out and maintain an optimum state in response to a wide variety of external challenges.

Simple rules underpin complex systems

An important but contested insight is that the capacity of systems to evolve to new patterns of order can arise from the recursive application of a relatively small number of simple rules. For example, the complex phenomenon of bird flocking or fish shoaling emerges from the recursive application of three simple rules: move to the centre of the crowd; maintain a minimum distance from your neighbour; and move at the speed of the element in front of you. The suggestion is that underpinning complex behaviour are a small number of simple rules or guiding principles.

Identifying the rules of a system through the use of observation or analysis of narrative and experimentation on a small scale can instigate change and reconfigure complex systems.[10]

Complexity theory and health economics

Admittedly, the economic literature is acknowledging that individuals seldom act as consistent rational actors but have unique non-linear interpretations of the world around them,[11] and chaos and complexity theory are already exerting an impact on mainstream economics.[12] Mannion and Small[13] have argued for the need to engage with the loss of general laws and the need to think more contingently within a post-modern framework where truths and knowledge are multiple, contingent, malleable and dynamic. There are a number of health

---

Box 30.3:   Feature of healthcare as an ecosystem

- A systems approach which focuses on interactions between parts and overall system performance.
- Individuals are locally free agents bound together by common principles and values.
- Individuals and institutions within an ecosystem coevolve.
- Ecosystems self-organise and are to be nutured rather than engineered.
- Individuals and institutions cooperate, exchange information and have good practice.

---

economists who argue for a breakout from the conventional neoclassical framework (in economic terminology, from a 'welfare' to an 'extra-welfare' perspective), but the majority remain grounded in the linear, reductionist method of analysis and decision making. For example, health economists continue to call for a more accurate measurement of the productivity of the NHS workforce with a view to inducing greater activity by incentive manipulation.[14]

Replacing the metaphor of a market for an ecosystem may be a useful first step (Box 30.3). Each element cannot be understood in isolation but interacts in an integrated system of coevolving elements. In the shifting topography of the health service, a change in one element alters the context for all other elements – all parts are adapting by learning to survive in an environment that is provided by coexisting parts. Ecosystems cannot be engineered – there are no causal links that promise sophisticated tools for analysing and predicting system behaviour. Rather than spend time on detailed planning and striving to calculate a solution by the continuous addition of rules and measurement, decision makers should be content with setting minimum specifications, establishing boundaries and letting the system settle into a condition that satisfies the constraints placed on it. How can these insights be applied to decision making? The trick is to match the approach with the complexity of the task as shown in Figure 30.1.

A rational approach underpinned by the principles of modern science is important in areas where there is likely to be a high degree of predictability and agreement among stakeholders about the level of predictability – for example, a decision based on the analysis of the costs and benefits of two competing blood pressure lowering drugs. However, much of healthcare decision making takes place within a network of non-linear interactions where there is uncertainty over how outputs can be measured and how inputs are converted to outputs. In such situations, complexity theory can facilitate an understanding of what creates patterns of order and behaviour and how these patterns

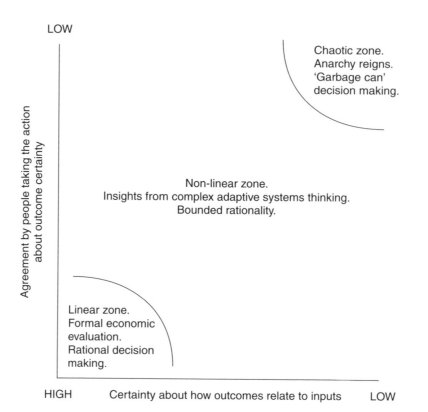

Figure 30.1:   Matching the analytical approach to the complexity of the task (after Stacey[7]).

emerge. As an example, the final section of this chapter will explore how complexity insights could be applied to the rationing agenda at the national level.

Insights into rationing from complex adaptive systems theory

Health care rationing is an area hedged with constraints, intermediate positions, arguments and counter arguments characterised by the common perception that healthcare is a linear, reductionist and deterministic system over which there is political and managerial control. International experience suggests that this may be wishful thinking and that rationing is inherently messy without any convergence to a common workable framework.

Some commentators have taken a counterview to health economists and argued that discretional rationing can respond more flexibly and sensitively to the heterogeneity of patients, doctors and their treatments.[16] Hunter[17] has argued that 'decision making in healthcare is an iterative process of "muddling through elegantly" from which a decision is arrived at'. Butler[18] argues that a sensitive and intelligent kind of muddling through seems to accord with the reality of how things are done at the coal face and argues that the discourses about what is right and what is feasible must keep in step with each other. Kline[19] sees policy making as experimental and incremental, an approach that may represent a more sophisticated and realistic form of rationality rather than attempts to devise technical fixes.

The evidence suggests that although citizens wish to be consulted, they do not want to make rational decisions directly,[20] are unable to reach agreement about general principles[21] and have preferences that can change with time.[22] This suggests that policy makers should act as agents for citizens, but that citizens should be involved in developing principles upon which these agents should act.[23] In summary, the current process of decision making can be conceptualised as a system of equivocation and paradox. Decisions are the result of a complex set of interactions in which there are a number of obstacles and a dilution of decisions resulting from attempts to avoid the disutility associated with denial in which all collude to minimise any distress arising from the responsibility for denying care.[24]

Although these commentators recognise the limitations of rational decision making within the model of modern science, they fail to set their commentaries within the context of a complexity frame of reference. What insights does non-linear systems thinking offer this agenda? First, no individual can make sense of the entire phenomena of healthcare. The realities of organisational life consist of all the details of all the events in the organisation's history as well as the actions of all their members. Second, we cannot analyse the system by reducing it into its component parts or escaping the conflict of values by retreating to an 'ideologically and organisationally simpler world'. Third, the source of standards is the previous history of the system itself. The system feeds back on itself rather than feeding back with reference to an external set point. Fourth, the emphasis should be on the interaction between stakeholders rather than their individual properties. Fifth, we need to recognise that these interactions are configured by power relationships.

An alternative approach to the rationing problem would be to recognise that the resources of complexity are best suited to the expression of complex problems through the reiterated and integrated judgement of a collection of stakeholders and experts. Their interactions would organise themselves with reference to themselves into emergent processes from which decisions can emerge as 'a shared moral sensitivity'.

From a practical perspective how would this model develop? The focus is on the priority setting process itself and the creation of the conditions for self-organisation underpinned by the recursive application of a small number of simple rules by relevant stakeholders from which a satisfactory solution will

---

Box 30.4:   Some 'simple rules' that could underpin emergent rationing

- To treat equals equally with due dignity, especially when near to death.
- To meet people's needs for healthcare as efficiently as possible (imposing the least sacrifice on others).
- To minimise inequalities in the lifetime health of the population.

---

emerge. Box 30.4 shows some possible simple rules suggested by health economist Alan Williams quoted in Hutton and Maynard[25] (although undoubtedly he would be alarmed to see them used in this context!).

An important factor in the success of this framework would be high levels of trust, a reduction of power differentials and a mutual understanding of each stakeholders' perspective against a background of organisations that are flexible enough to adapt, creative enough to innovate and responsive enough to learn. Perhaps to put it more simply, if you look after the interactions, the outcomes will look after themselves.

Rationing as an emergent phenomena in a non-linear system reflects a pragmatic approach that is already in place – a model that reflects reality rather than attempting to force it into a disciplinary framework. For example, the National Institute for Clinical Excellence (NICE) through the synthesis of all available evidence reaches 'a judgement as to whether on balance an intervention can be recommended as a cost effective use of NHS resources'.[26]

Self-organised criticality is a law of complex systems that allows them to optimise their efficiency as they learn and evolve with time.[27] In essence, the trick for the rationing agenda is to facilitate the interaction of relevant stakeholders in a rich conversation within a framework that emphasises the importance of high trust and egalitarian relationships underpinned by transparent simple rules. If the system is maintained at a level of self-organised criticality, solutions will emerge that are satisfactory and which provide a platform for the whole process to start again.

Conclusion

It seems we live in two worlds: one created by nature with its capacity to innovate and adapt, the other built by humans – often rigid, inefficient and incapable of delivering what we want. Drawing on insights from nature challenges the linear formulation of modern science and recognises a world where many phenomena are directed by the complex non-linear interactions of many parts – interactions that cannot always be understood by breaking systems down into their constituent elements and the application of analytical rules. In many areas, the clockwork universe may finally be running down.

Complexity science sees disciplines as disparate as economics, business, meteorology, ecology, politics and medicine converging to similar themes. Viewing health economics through the model of a non-linear multidimensional phase space can accommodate the neoclassical model with the pursuit of non-economic goals such as approval, status and compassion while recognising that all action is socially situated and cannot be explained by individual motives alone. Unfortunately, unlike some of their mainstream economic colleagues, health economists seem slow to recognise the potential.

Recognising healthcare organisations as non-linear systems challenges a number of traditional notions, but offers us useful insights for future development. It cautions against the use of information derived from history or present day data that may not improve the ability to predict subsequent events. It emphasises the need to learn by reflection on the difference between rhetoric and experienced reality, forcing us to rethink our ideas on causation and intervention. In many cases, outcomes are often not an optimal solution to a problem, but a learning that leads to a decision to take certain actions in the knowledge that this will lead in general not to the problem being solved but to a new situation in which the whole process can begin again. It recognises that evidence is contextual, subjective and limited and offers us a philosophical and metaphorical bridge to reality. Emphasising the importance of narrative it suggests that qualitative methods can provide better descriptive, explanatory and predictive models to achieve a satisfactory way forward in many areas of healthcare decision making.

If nothing else, complexity theory alerts us to the fact that there are no quick policy fixes or any easy way to integrate analytical techniques to participatory processes. Over 60 years ago, the economist Keynes (as cited by Mannion and Small[28]) suggested that 'we need to invent wisdom for a new age and that in the meantime, we must appear unorthodox, troublesome and dangerous'. The science of complex adaptive systems may be this new wisdom that we seek. Alternatively, it may just be a passing fad merely articulating common sense and emphasising that we should all be nice to each other. What is irrefutable is that the dominance of linear orthodoxy has been challenged. Health economists would be wise to take note.

References

1   Black N (2001) Evidence based policy: proceed with care. *BMJ.* **323**: 275–9.
2   Kernick DP (1998) Has health economics lost its way. *BMJ.* **317**: 197–9.

3   Holm S (1998) Goodbye to the simple solutions: the second phase of priority setting in healthcare. *BMJ*. **317**: 1000–2.

4   Mannion R and Goddard M (2001) Impact of published clinical outcomes data: case study in a NHS hospital trust. *BMJ*. **323**: 260–3.

5   Hayes B and Haines A (1998) Barriers and bridges to evidence based clinical practice. *BMJ*. **317**: 273–6.

6   Cilliers P (1998) *Complexity and Postmodernism*. Routledge Press, London.

7   Stacey R (2000) *Strategic Management and Organisational Dynamics: the challenge of complexity*. Pearson Education, London.

8   Greenberg D (1997) NIH resists research funding linked to patient load. *Lancet*. **349**: 1229.

9   Department of Health (1998) *The Health of the Nation: a policy assessed*. HMSO, London.

10 Plsek P (2001) Re-designing healthcare with insights from the science of complex adaptive systems. In: *Crossing the Quality Chasm: a new health system for the 21st century*. National Academy Press, Washington DC, 329–35.

11 Ormerod P (2000) *Butterfly Economics*. Panthion Books, New York.

12 Benhabib J (1992) *Cycles and Chaos in Economic Equilibrium*. Princeton University Press, Princeton.

13 Mannion R and Small N (1999) Post-modern health economics. *Health Care Analysis*. **7**: 255–72.

14 Bloor K and Maynard A (2001) Workforce productivity and incentive structures in the UK National Health Service. *J Health Serv Res Policy*. **6**: 5–113.

15 Royston G and Dick P (1998) Healthcare ecology. *Br J Healthcare Management*. **4(5)**: 238–41.

16 Machanic D (1995) Dilemmas in rationing healthcare services: the case for implicit rationing. *BMJ*. **310**: 1655–9.

17 Hunter D (1997) *Desperately Seeking Solutions*. Longman, London.

18 Butler J (1999) *The Ethics of Healthcare Rationing: principals and practices*. Cassell, London.

19 Kline R (1998) Puzzling out priorities. *BMJ*. **318**: 959–60.

20 Kneeshaw J (1997) What does the public think about rationing? A review of the evidence in rationing. In: B New (ed) *Talk and Action in Healthcare*. BMJ Publishing, London, 58–76.

21 Cuadras-Morato L and Pinto-Prades J (2001) Equity considerations in health care: the relevance of claims. *Health Economics*. **10**: 187–205.

22 Shiell A, Seymour J, Hawe P *et al.* (2000) Are preferences over health states complete? *Health Economics*. **9**: 47–55.

23 Mooney G (1998) Communitarian claims as an ethical basis for allocating health care resources. *Soc Sci Med*. **49(9)**: 1171–80.

24 Coast J (2001) Citizens, their agents and health care rationing: an exploratory study using qualitative methods. *Health Economics*. **10**: 159–74.

25 Hutton J and Maynard A (2000) A NICE challenge for health economists. *Health Economics*. **9**: 89–93.

26 National Institute for Clinical Excellence (1999) *An Appraisal of New and Existing Technology: interim guidance for manufacturers and sponsors*. NICE, London.

27 Bak P (1996) *How Nature Works: the science of self organised criticality*. Springer-Verlag, New York.

28 Mannion R and Small N (1999) Post-modern health economics. *Health Care Analysis*. **7**: 255–72.

CHAPTER 31

Health economics: continuing imperialism?

Alan Maynard

Introduction

The subdiscipline of health economics is inevitably imperialistic with its devotees continuing to argue that the problems it addresses are ubiquitous and the economics 'tool kit' has universal application. As one practitioner of these darks forces, Alan Williams, has argued, 'be reasonable, do it my way!'.[1] It is curious that such sensible pleas for rationality and reasonableness fall on so many deaf ears among 'operatives' in the healthcare industry!

The nature of the economic approach to the production of health (an outcome desired by patients) and healthcare (an activity which hopefully contributes to the health of patients, and always contributes to the income of providers!) is dealt with in the first part of this chapter. The next part addresses the issue of why health economics and the creation of economics-based medicine grows in influence slowly but inexorably, continually opposed by Luddites and commercial interests who feel, sometimes totally erroneously, threatened by the wisdom of the health economics tribe!

The nature of health economics

The objective of investment in healthcare is to produce health, although you would never guess this from the way practitioners and managers fail to evaluate changes in the health status of individual patients and the population! These folk typically organise their lives and their careers around issues of spending (inputs) and processes (activity in terms of patients treated and waiting times targets).

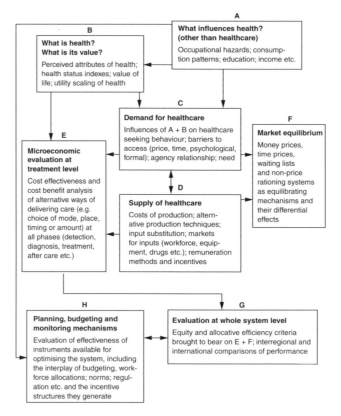

Figure 31.1: The nature of health economics.

The nature of health economics is summarised in Figure 31.1. The primary focus of concern is box B – the measurement and valuation of health. There are many determinants of health (box A), and in countries such as Brazil spending on the education of young women on techniques of oral rehydration and food programmes targeting poor children give more health gain than spending on healthcare.

The microeconomics of healthcare (boxes C, D, E and F) is the area where most health economists earn their crusts! The most rewarding activity (in a pecuniary sense!) for economists is investment in and practice in micro-economic evaluation at the treatment level. By riding on the coat tails of medical practitioners and the pharmaceutical industry, this subspecies of the economics tribe have made themselves useful emphasising that the evaluation of the clin-ical effectiveness of competing diagnostic and therapeutic interventions is a necessary but not a sufficient condition to achieve an efficient use of society's scarce healthcare resources in the healthcare system. These folk have empha-sised that healthcare rationing is ubiquitous; doctors are paid high salaries (relative to non-clinical professors!) to deprive (or simply not offer) patients of care which would benefit them and which they want. Such difficult professional choices are best based on evidence. Thus the evidence-based medicine (EBM) 'brigade' led by Sackett and other medical Messiahs, promulgated the gospel of practicing in relation to what was known about clinical effectiveness – if the intervention can be shown to 'work', lets use it! While this approach inevitably prompts speculation about what doctors did before EBM (e.g. toss coins to determine clinical activity perhaps?), as it manifested itself in the Cochrane Collaboration and the Scottish Intercollegiate Guidelines Network (SIGN) it was very useful.[2]

However it was of course incomplete; lots of interventions 'work' but with limited budgets we can afford only some of them. What prioritisation principles should be used to determine which of the many interventions that 'work' should be funded and provided to the many patients competing for care? Any choice which determines who is treated should be informed by the value of what is gained (i.e. improvements in health status) and what is given (the opportunity cost of the intervention). Only if both costs and benefit are estimated and used to rank competing interventions, can resources be targeted in such a way as to maximise the impact of the cash limited NHS budget (£50 billion) on the health of the British population.[3,4]

Of course, this preference for efficiency (maximising the health gains produced at least cost) may not be shared by society. For instance, doctors are allowed to practice inefficiently and keep low birth weight babies alive presumably because society values such lives more highly than those of middle and old age customers of the NHS who are, as a consequence, required to queue for cost effective interventions such as hip replacements and cataract removals. Such equity judgements should be explicit so the implications of these choices are explicit and those practising inefficiently can be made accountable to their paymasters.

Thus the artisans working in box E (*see* Figure 31.1) have to deal with the establishment of rationing or prioritisation criteria and the complex processes of identifying, measuring and valuing the costs and benefits of competing interventions. However, this work is now seen as much broader than it was 10 years ago because of the recognition of the obstacles to translating evidence into practice. Thus microeconomic evaluation techniques can be used also to appraise the costs and benefits of, for instance, competing financial and non-financial incentive systems.

Boxes C, D and E in the figure are core economics activities where health economists have not been as active as they might have been. For instance, there is a labour economics 'tool kit' which has not been deployed extensively in healthcare in Britain. Work on the economic determinants of the supply of labour could produce results central to improving the performance of the NHS, especially when in the short-term labour supply is relatively fixed until medical school and other training investments bear fruit. Thus is it cost effective to substitute nurses for GPs?[5] Are wages the primary determinant of nurse labour supply? There is evidence that it is not.[6] How can economists inform the reform of the consultant and the GP contract of employment? The economics literature on team working and performance incentives shows that neither of these much-advocated incentive mechanisms are efficient.[6,7]

Boxes G and H deal with issues of macro-system importance. They highlight the issue of health reform as social experimentation. Doctors, nurses and drug companies are told they must practice EBM and be much more accountable for their performance. Yet politicians worldwide can wake up this morning with a reform 'wheeze' in their mind and implement it if their civil servants are as efficient as those in Whitehall village. Of course such 'redisorganisations' of the NHS change the organisational structure, but appear to have all too little impact on practitioners. For example, the average productivity for GPs and consultants, crudely measured with the poor available data, appears to have been constant for decades despite continued reforms by Tory and Labour ministers.[8] The central policy and research issue, as ever, is that such social experiments should be evaluated in just the same way as a new drug or a new surgical procedure. Politicians can destroy patient health just as easily as doctors can by failing to adopt economics/evidence-based policies.

Each of the boxes in Figure 31.1 are interrelated and feed into one another. For instance, the work on evaluation at the treatment level is dependent on good measures of population health. While robust and valid measures of health related quality of life have been developed and used in hundreds of clinical trials, it remains remarkable that these have not been used routinely to measure.[9,10]

The growth of health economics

Health economics, both as a subdiscipline, and as an influence on health and healthcare policy, has grown slowly over three decades. Initially focused at Aberdeen (Health Economics Research Unit), Brunel and York (Centre for Health Economics), it is now well established also in places such as Bristol, East Anglia and Sheffield. This growth has been led by highly focused and determined individuals (e.g. Alan Williams at York[1]) and research centres and training activies which have populated the current units in the UK and abroad with York and Aberdeen practitioners, or 'mafia'!

However, these supply side efforts alone would not have succeeded if there had been no demand for health economists. This demand initially came from distinguished medical practitioners who see the logic of the economic approach to healthcare. Thus Archie Cochrane's famous book reflected economic thinking because of the influence on the author of Alan Williams.[2,11] Williams was also influential with a Chief Scientist in the Department of Health, Sir Douglas Black, who was persuaded to fund the York MSc. course in health economics.

During the 1970s and the 1980s, the growth in the awareness of clinical researchers of the need to ensure trials included economic elements, led to a growing market for health economists. By the end of the 1980s even the conservative Medical Research Council had established a Health Services Research Committee to fund such trials. In the early 1990s the EBM initiatives drew further funding into R&D and the demand for economics increased further.

However the 'revolution' is incomplete. The economists remain only modestly influential in determining the R&D agenda. While the investment in the area of the microeconomic evaluation of treatments continues to create most employment for economists in both the public and private sectors (the pharmaceutical industry),[12] there remains much to be done in applying economics techniques to the labour and capital markets (e.g. is the private finance initiative efficient?[12]) and in regulation. Research funding in these areas is very modest and, as a consequence, policy continues to be 'unconfused' by evidence!

Why is there this lack of investment? One reason is the economic ignorance of many policy makers and practitioners in the healthcare sector. Such people often appear to prefer opinion, particularly if it reinforces their prejudices and does not disturb the distribution of incomes, jobs and power on which they depend. As the fictitious Sir Humphrey Appleby argued in the BBC TV series *Yes Minister*, ' it is folly to undermine authority with evidence'!

Another problem is the supply of health economists. With this profession being successful in creating bodies such as the National Institute for Clinical Excellence (NICE), the demand for health economists in the drug industry and academia has increased sharply. However, there is no increased funding of training such people by either the public or private sectors.

Without doubt, economics-based medicine can be threatening. If NICE decrees a new drug should be adopted on the basis of clinical and cost effectiveness, its funding has an opportunity cost – less resource is available for hip replacements and other waiting time policies. The adoption of NICE advice on hip prostheses and ENT guidelines, if applied disturb existing practices and power relationships – all change, even if it brings greater efficiency, is redistributive and losers in such processes tend to 'shout' louder than gainers!

Conclusions

The economics tribe will not go away and their influence at both the micro-treatment and macro-system levels of policy making are bound to grow as the NHS is driven towards the new EBM: economics-based medicine! However, economists have to be modest. While their contribution to creating health and a more efficient and equitable healthcare system is considerable, it can only come to full fruition if research is collaborative with other disciplines and development or the translation of evidence into practice is well coordinated with power barons in Whitehall and the professional mafias!

References

1 Williams A (1997) *Being Reasonable about the Economics of Health: selected essays of Alan Williams.* Compiled and edited by AJ Culyer and Alan Maynard. Edward Elgar, Cheltenham.

2 Maynard A and Chalmers I (eds) (1997) *Non Random Reflections on Health Services Research: on the 25th anniversary of Archie Cochrane's effectiveness and efficiency.* BMJ Publishing, London.

3 Maynard A (1997) Evidence based medicine: an incomplete method for informing treatment choices. *Lancet.* **349**: 126–8.

4 Cookson R, Mcdaid D and Maynard A (2001) Wrong SIGN NICE mess: is national guidance distorting the allocation of resources? *BMJ.* **323**: 743–5.

5 Richardson G, Maynard A, Cullum N and Kindig D (1997) Skill mix changes: substitution or service development. *Health Policy.* **45**: 119–32.

6 Maynard A and Bloor K (2001) Reforming the contract for UK consultants. *BMJ.* **322**: 541–3.

7 Ratto M with Burgess S, Croxson B, Jewitt I and Propper C (2001) *Team-based Incentives in the NHS: an economic analysis. Working Paper 01/37.* Centre for Market and Public Organisation, Department of Economics, University of Bristol.

8 Bloor K and Maynard A (2001) Workforce productivity and incentive structure in the UK NHS. *J Health Services Res Policy.* **6(2)**: 105–13.

9 Brooks R and the EuroQol group (1996) Euro-Qol: the current state of play. *Health Policy.* **37**: 53–72.

10 Maynard A (In press) Economic aspects of clinical governance. In: J Thompson and S Pickering (eds) *The Practice of Clinical Governance.* Routledge, London.

11 Cochrane AL (1972) *Efficiency and Effectiveness: random reflections on health services research.* Nuffield Provincial Hospitals Trust, London.

12 Maynard A and Kanavos P (2000) Health economics: an evolving paradigm. *Health Economics.* **9(3)**: 183–90.

Epilogue

Well, there it is. What started off as an introductory text has got rather out of control but, hopefully, readers aren't more confused at the end than at the beginning of this book. The aim has been to demonstrate some of the important insights and techniques that health economics can offer with its emphasis on explicit and rational frameworks to facilitate the efficient distribution of limited healthcare resources. I would value any comments, advice or suggestions for a second edition of this book. We have seen that there are many concerns and that the impact of health economics to date has been limited. A number of health economists have responded with a call for a retreat to academia and disciplinary basics but are they in danger of isolating themselves from the real world?

A paradigm is a set of received beliefs in a subject area. A discipline agrees on a framework of shared assumptions which are strengthened by education, language and professional association. These assumptions exert a deep hold on the scientific mind, and what follows is a strenuous and devoted attempt to force nature into the conceptual boxes that have been supplied. Health economists remain within a paradigm characterised by a linear view of the world underpinned by the fundamental axioms of a market model and rational consumer behaviour. This is a model that may not always be in step with the contingencies of the real world of healthcare, which explains why the impact of health economics has not been commensurate with its academic effort. Where should the discipline go from here?

First, it must recognise that the majority of health economic discourse is totally opaque to end users of economic information. Policy makers cannot be expected to draw on insights from inaccessible models constructed on esoteric debate and abstruse mathematics. As there is little or no knowledge of even the most basic economic theory among decision makers, perhaps the first priority should be a refocusing of effort into presentation of its concepts and education of its principles.

Second, health economists should move away from their dominant linear mode of thinking – the belief that complex systems can be understood by an analysis of their component parts and the predictable interactions between them. This approach is often at odds with the providers of healthcare who live in a complex environment and who seek generic predictions of trends rather than exact solutions. The need is to balance evidence, economics, equity and patient empowerment within a non-linear system of multiple constraints and limited room for manoeuvre.

To this end, health economists should work more closely with other disciplines and the decision makers whom they seek to influence rather than offering prescriptions from outside the healthcare environment. They should move away from institutionalised theory that practitioners and managers are expected to apply and which invariably bears no relationship to their requirements for pragmatic strategies.

There are those who are less generous of the whole economic programme and claim that economics is what economists do, and what economists do is study questions that can be handled with their own expertise. Who would suggest that health economists will continue to look for the conditions and translations that let their theory survive however ludicrous they may be, rather than admit to failure; that citizens evolve systems of production and distribution without economic models; that what motivates us is not utility but to see meaning through the relationships we have with each other; that the focus should be on what has happened and what actions may have served us better rather than generalisable frameworks of prediction and control.

Nevertheless, health economists are not going to go away and can offer important insights and techniques to facilitate the commissioning and delivery of efficient and equitable healthcare. The theoretical framework needs to be grounded more appropriately in the everyday experience of those engaging with healthcare systems in a world that is socially constructed but which can accommodate goal seeking behaviour.

Health economists have an important role in facilitating the distribution of society's limited resources, but need to move on from their obsessions with methodological purity and guideline refinement; to open a conversation with those they seek to influence; to think more contingently – perhaps concentrating on being vaguely right rather than arguing among themselves how to be precisely wrong.

David Kernick
St Thomas Health Centre
Cowick Street
Exeter EX4 1HJ
email: su1838@eclipse.co.uk

Glossary

Clinical governance
A framework through which NHS organisations are accountable for continuously improving the quality of their services and safeguarding high standards of care by creating an environment in which excellence in clinical care will flourish.

Commissioning
The arrangements that link purchasers and providers. These include basic requirements such as price structure and the clarification of organisational objectives through to the monitoring of contractual relationships and the termination or renegotiation of contracts.

Complex systems
A system of individual agents, who have the freedom to act in ways that are not always predictable, and whose actions are interconnected such that one agent's actions changes the context for other agents. The interaction between agents is invariable non-linear.

Contingent valuation
A method of placing a monetary value (shadow price) on an item or attribute that is not available in a market by determining the maximum people who would be prepared to pay for it or the minimum they would be willing to accept to part with it.

Contract
A formal agreement between purchasers and providers that specifies what services will be provided and the terms on which they will be provided.

Cost benefit analysis
An economic analysis where all outcomes are valued in monetary units. Rarely used due to methodological problems in valuing all outcomes in monetary terms.

Cost consequences analysis
An economic analysis where costs and outcomes are presented in a disaggregated form rather than a single measure. Although this approach is not a

formal method of economic analysis, it is one that may be more attractive to decision makers who can apply their own weight to the various outcomes.

Cost effectiveness analysis
An economic analysis to compare interventions that have a common health outcome (e.g. reduction in blood pressure, life years saved).

Cost effectiveness ratio
The additional cost of obtaining a health effect from a given intervention when compared with a comparitor:

> i.e. (cost of intervention − cost alternative)/(benefit of intervention − benefit of alternative).

Cost minimisation analysis
An economic analysis where the consequences of two or more interventions being compared are equivalent. The analysis, therefore, focuses on costs alone, although the evidence of equivalent outcomes should be established prior to consideration of costs.

Cost of illness study
An exercise that attempts to quantify the burden of an illness by measuring all its costs in monetary terms.

Costs
An economic opportunity foregone. Costs can be direct costs whereby costs are associated directly with a healthcare intervention (e.g. GP salaries, drug costs) or indirect costs whereby costs are associated with reduced productivity due to illness, disability or death.

Cost utility analysis
An economic analysis where outcomes are valued on individual preferences (e.g. quality adjusted life years gained). Although this approach is gaining in importance due to the need to compare different interventions at a national level, many methodological problems remain.

Decision tree
An analytical framework representing choices available, outcomes of those choices and probabilities of achieving those outcomes. Decision trees can be used to improve decision making and illuminate the data that are required to make a decision.

Disability adjusted life years
A measure used to establish the burden of a disease or to compare outcomes of different interventions. It combines the expected length of life lost with the adjusted number of years lived with the disability.

Discounting
Cost may be incurred and benefits enjoyed at different times when comparing interventions. As we prefer to incur our benefits sooner and costs later, these variables must be multiplied by a factor so that they can be evaluated and compared within the same time frame. This is known as discounting and is usually applied to economic trials that last for more than a year.

Economic evaluation
A comparative analysis of alternative courses of action in terms of both their costs and consequences and the values attached to them.

Economic model
The fundamental starting point of economic theory is that the best way of distributing society's limited resources is using the model of a competitive market where decisions are determined by independent consumers and producers using signals in the form of prices regulated by the interplay of supply and demand. Consumers behave in such a way as to maximise their utility or well being.

Economics
The study of how society allocates its scarce resources.

Efficiency
Ensuring that goods and services are allocated so as to maximise the welfare of the community. In general, this is obtained either by achieving a given output from the minimum possible input or producing the maximum possible from a fixed resource. Efficiency advocates the adoption of two basic principles: ensure that sacrifices entailed are kept to a minimum and make sure that no activity is pursued unless the benefits gained outweigh the benefits foregone.

Equity
Fairness in allocating limited resources. A contested concept but generally agreed to infer that patients should be treated equally irrespective of age, sex or socioeconomic status and those with greater need should receive preferential treatment.

Governance
The institutions, rules, regulations and protocols that govern stakeholders in undertaking transactions.

Health
Subject to wide individual, social and cultural interpretations. It may include for example: the absence of disease, pain or distress; a state of complete physical, mental and social well being; a set of basic conditions which enable a person to fulfil their realistic, chosen and biological potentials.

Health economics
The discipline of economics applied to the topic of health. Both the philosophical and methodological bases of health economics are, as a result, founded on their similar bases in economics.

Health technology
Any method used by those working in health services to promote health, screen, diagnose and treat disease, and improve rehabilitation and long-term care.

Health technology assessment
Considers the effectiveness, appropriateness, cost and broader implications of technologies using both primary research and systematic review. It seeks to meet the information needs of those who manage and provide care.

Marginal analysis
Because the relationship between costs and benefits is rarely proportional (not a straight line), the important measurement is not an average cost per benefit (the total cost divided by the total benefit), but the incremental ratio (how increments in benefit change with increments in costs.) This is known as a marginal analysis.

Marginal cost
The extra cost of one extra unit of service provided.

Market
Any arrangement by which buyers and sellers come together. It may be a physical location or virtual (e.g. stock markets). An internal or quasi market is the term coined for market-type arrangements that were introduced to the public sector during the 1990s. A managed market is the term used to refer to markets that are subject to regulation in order to make sure that important social objectives (e.g. fairness) are not neglected.

Mixed economy
The collection of arrangements involving the public and independent sectors for the provision, purchasing and governance of specific services.

Needs
A contested concept with a number of interpretations. Perhaps the most common is – what agents sanctioned by society (traditionally healthcare professionals) think will benefit population or patients' health. Needs contrast with wants – what patients think will benefit their health.

NICE
The National Institute for Clinical Excellence (NICE) which was set up in April 1999 to 'enable evidence of clinical and cost effectiveness to be integrated to inform a national judgement on the value of a treatment(s) relative to alternative uses of the resources' and thereby provide 'guidance on whether a treatment (new or existing) can be recommended for routine use in the NHS (in England and Wales)'.

Non-linearity
Small changes can have large system effects, large effects can lead to small system changes. Non-linear systems are sensitive to initial conditions and cannot be understood by reduction into their component parts – the whole is different from the sum of the parts.

Normative or welfare economics
A branch of economics that uses economics to facilitate decision making from the perspective of making the most efficient use of limited resources. It assumes that the welfare of society is equal to the sum of the welfare of the individuals within it. The practical expression of this search for efficiency in healthcare is the conduct of economic evaluation.

Opportunity cost
An approach that views cost as a sacrifice rather than financial expenditure – a benefit foregone. The opportunity cost is the value of the next best alternative use of the resources under consideration. Unlike accountancy there is more to costs than the spending of money.

Perspective
The viewpoint of an economic study. The perspective will determine which costs and benefits to quantify. For example, the viewpoint could be a societal, NHS, primary care group, GP practice or patient perspective. Different perspectives may give different answers.

Pharmacoeconomics
The application of health economics to medicines, drawing on the same techniques.

Principals and agents
In all but the least complicated of economic systems, it is necessary for an individual or organisation (the principal) to delegate some activities to an agent, who is expected to accomplish these activities at the principal's behest.

Programme budgeting and marginal analysis (PBMA)
A tool developed by economists to provide a framework for decision makers to incorporate evidence of effectiveness and cost effectiveness, as well as other criteria such as equity of access. PBMA recognises that decision makers are not starting with a blank sheet of paper to design ideal solutions. Hence, it involves examining the existing allocation of resources to a programme and examining alternative (usually resource neutral) ways of allocating those resources.

Positive or explanatory economics
A branch of economics that uses economic theory to explain and predict the operation of the economic system.

Quality adjusted life year (QALY)
An outcome measure that encompasses both quality and quantity of life. Its advantage is that it allows disparate health interventions to be compared.

Quality of life
A highly contested concept. Perhaps the most succinct definition is the gap between experience and expectation.

Rationing
The need to distribute healthcare under conditions where everyone cannot receive the healthcare from which they would benefit. Explicit rationing is when distribution is based on defined rules of entitlement. Implicit rationing is when it is the discretion of gatekeepers that determines access into the system (for example GPs).

Sensitivity analysis
A technique that allows the outcome of an economic analysis to be tested over a range of situations likely to be found in practice to determine the robustness of analysis to potential changes in key variables.

Standard gamble
A method to calculate the utility of an intervention by asking individuals to choose between living the rest of their lives in their current state or gambling on a cure which if won will mean perfect health and if lost, signify death.

Systematic review
A review of the evidence on a clearly formulated question that uses systematic and explicit methods to identify, select and critically appraise relevant primary research, and to extract and analyse data from the studies that are included in the review.

Time trade-off
A method to determine the utility of an intervention that asks subjects to decide how many years of remaining life they would exchange for complete health.

Transaction
The interactions and connections between purchasers and providers.

Transaction costs
The costs incurred in buying and selling goods and services.

Utility
In economic theory, utility signifies the benefit a person expects to gain from the consumption of goods or services – an indicator of the consumer's strength of preference. Utility is an attribute that motivates us to choose one action over another. It will be a complex function of a number of elements that might include physical, psychological and moral components that we integrate in our minds to form preferences. In health economics, utility is seen as the value an individual places on a health state. Ideally, this value is obtained by finding what a subject is prepared to sacrifice to obtain a health state.

Useful resources

Cost information

Unit Costs of Health and Social Care

www.ukc.ac.uk/pssru
The most comprehensive and accurate compendium of cost data in the NHS is published by the Personal Social Services Research Unit. It brings together estimates and underlying methodology of national unit costs of health and social care services. Essential reading for those involved in providing or evaluating care or undertaking cost research.

The NHS Costing Manual (Department of Health)

www.doh.gov.uk/nhsexec/costing/htm (not for the faint hearted)
The Government manual which sets out the principles and practice of costing to be applied in the NHS which underpins the production of the national schedule of reference costs.

The Reference Cost Schedule

www.doh.gov.uk/nhsexec/refcosts.htm
Estimates of NHS costs based on costs provided by suppliers. Thought by many to be largely fictional.

Databases of economic studies

The NHS Economic Evaluation Database

www.york.ac.uk/nhsdhp
A comprehensive database of all economic evaluations that are published.

Useful information

The Centre for Health Economics, University of York

www.york.ac.uk/inst/che
The epicentre for health economics in the UK provides a useful starting point for courses, training, journals and other links.

The Office of Health Economics

www.ohe.org
Supported and founded by the Association of British Pharmaceutical Industry, the OHE publishes a number of useful publications. Of particular note is its compendium of health statistics. This is probably the most comprehensive collection of UK health statistics and is published annually. Although it is not available to download it can be found in most libraries.

The Health Policy and Economic Research Unit of the BMA

www.bma.org.uk/policy
Contains a wide variety of economic and statistical information and analysis most of which can be downloaded.

The BMJ Health Economics Collection

www.bmj.com/cgi/collection/health_economics
Full text of all health economic publications from the BMJ. Useful to get a feel of the subject from the perspective of a general readership.

The Department of Health website

www.doh.gov.uk
Gives a large number of useful links particularly in research and development. Interesting data in the link to the National Institute for Statistics.

The NHS Health Technology Assessment Programme

www.ncchta.org
Contains some excellent monographs on areas of health economics that are considered in some depth but remain accessible. Can be downloaded directly from the web.

The National Institute for Clinical Excellence

www.nice.org.uk
An explicit (well almost) review of the work of the National Institute for Clinical Excellence (NICE).

Bandolier

www.jr2.ox.ac.uk/bandolier
Some accessible and relevant economic evaluations.

PubMed

www.pubmedcentral.nih.gov
Get abstracts of your journal references here.

Omni

omni.ac.uk
A gateway to evaluated Internet resources in health and medicine.

National electronic Library for Health

www.nelh.nhs.uk
The NHS gateway to healthcare information.

Appendix 1: Studies assessing the impact and relevance of health economic analyses in practice at purchaser level

Author(s) and publication date	Scale and scope	Research focus	Methods and sources	Findings
McNamee, Godber (1995)[1]	Evaluation of 'Purchaser Intelligence Pilot' which provided health economic input into decision making, primarily in two English HAs	Factors contributing to success (where 'success' is not defined explicitly)	Researchers' personal experiences and impressions gained as those involved in the provision of 'intelligence'	Barriers included deficiencies in data on evidence, cost and activity, the lack of a systematic approach to decision making in purchasing organisations
Harrison (1996)[2]	Evaluation of 'Purchaser Intelligence Pilot' (see above)	Outputs in terms of policy relevance/ implementability Outcomes in terms of changing contract patterns and less tangible spin-offs	Interviews, documents, correspondence, expert opinion	Barriers to implementation included weak purchaser legitimacy and differences in perspectives in terms of (a) the way in which effectiveness should be conceived (e.g. GPs may value interventions which reduce pressure on them), (b) what constitutes 'evidence' (c) what constitutes 'cost'
Drummond, Cooke, Walley (1996)[3] Drummond, Walley (1997)[4] Walley, Barton, Cooke, Drummond (1997)[5]	Survey of all prescribing advisers and directors of public health at commissioner level in England, Scotland and Wales (hospital pharmacists also surveyed)	Investigation of perceived barriers to the use of economic evaluation in relation to drug therapy	Questionnaires	Barriers include the multiple objectives being pursued by decision makers, difficulties disinvesting from services and concerns about the validity of economic evaluations

Study	Sample	Focus	Method	Findings
Miller, Vale (1997)[6]	Key decision makers in one English HA (n = 12) and one Scottish Health Board (n = 17)	Purchaser attitudes to the use of programme budgeting and marginal analysis	Interviews	Decision makers are not actively using health economic techniques. Barriers include the reactive nature of decision making, weak legitimacy on the part of purchaser organisations
Green (1998) (unpublished ScHARR report)[7]	Observations and findings from the development of marginal analysis in one HA	Barriers contributing to the failure to develop a full marginal analysis process	Observation	Barriers included lack of time and commitment, a failure to drive the process from the top and a failure to incorporate the priority setting exercise into mainstream organisational business
Duthie, Trueman, Chancellor, Diez (1999)[8]	Sample of decision makers (n = 34, HA staff = 6) from all over England (included GPs and hospital staff)	Relevance of health economic studies to decision makers	Interviews	Economists need to demonstrate better understanding of the NHS decision-making context so that arguments presented in studies are more relevant. GPs and HAs had different views about the relative importance of factors such as costs, patient satisfaction, quality of life issues and evidence. The fundamental premise of willingness-to-pay studies was challenged by most participants

Author(s) and publication date	Scale and scope	Research focus	Methods and sources	Findings
Hoffman, von der Schulenburg (2000)[9]	Sample of decision makers from nine EU countries	Attitudes of decision makers to economic evaluation studies (includes relevance, barriers, actual and potential use of studies)	Focus groups and interviews (for UK sample)	Results of economic evaluation studies are not widely used in decision making. Barriers include inflexible financial regimens, lack of credibility and perceived lack of practical relevance of studies
Stoykova, Drummond, Hoffman, Nixon, Glanville[10]	Sample of decision makers from two health authorities	Attitudes of decision makers to economic evaluation studies (includes relevance, barriers, actual and potential use of studies)	Focus groups (initial and follow-up)	'The main perceived limitation was that most published studies explored the cost effectiveness of particular health technologies and not broader health programmes, thus being of limited use to a decision maker at health authority level ... The limited generalisability of some economic evaluations was also identified as a significant disadvantage.'

References

1   McNamee P and Godber E (1995) *Assessing and Applying Effectiveness and Cost-effectiveness Evidence in Purchasing Organisations: problems and prospects.* Paper presented to the Health Economics Study Group, Aberdeen.

2   Harrison S (1996) *Northern and Yorkshire Regional Health Authority Purchasing Intelligence Project: an evaluation study.* NHS Executive (Northern and Yorkshire) and Nuffield Institute for Health, University of Leeds, Leeds.

3   Drummond M, Cooke J and Walley T (1996) *Economic Evaluation in Health Care Decision Making: evidence from the UK.* University of York Discussion Paper 148.

4   Drummond MCJ and Walley T (1997) Economic evaluation under managed competition: evidence from the UK. *Social Science Medicine.* **45(4):** 583–95.

5   Walley T *et al.* (1997) Economic evaluations of drug therapy: attitudes of primary care prescribing advisers in Great Britain. *Health Policy.* **41:** 61–72.

6   Miller L and Vale P (1997) *A Synthesis of Two Independent Surveys of Purchaser Views on the Use of Programme Budgeting and Marginal Analysis. Evidence of the need for national guidance?* HESG Paper.

7   Green C (1998) *Marginal Analysis: experiences in Rotherham.* ScHARR unpublished working paper. ScHARR, Sheffield.

8   Duthie T *et al.* (1999) Research into the use of health economics in decision making in the United Kingdom – Phase II. Is health economics 'for good or evil'? *Health Policy.* **46:** 143–57.

9   Hoffman C and von der Schulenburg J-M on behalf of the EUROMET group (2000) The influence of economic evaluation studies on decision making. A European survey. *Health Policy.* **52:** 179–92.

10 Stoykova B, Drummond M, Hoffman C, Nixon J and Glanville J (2000) *The Usefulness and Limitations of Published Economic Evaluations for NHS Decision-making.* Paper presented at HESG meeting, Nottingham, July 2000.

Appendix 2: PBMA or MA studies at local level in the NHS

Author(s) and publication date	Study setting	Study focus	Outcomes/outputs in terms of policy process reported
Donaldson, Farrar (1993)[1]	One Scottish Health Board	Dementia services	No information provided
Cohen (1994)[2] Cohen (1995)[3]	One Welsh HA	Multiprogramme approach initially. Main focus on maternal and early child health services	Yes. Agreement to incorporate findings into strategy documents and contracts
Lockett, Raftery, Richards (1995)[4]	One English HA	Macro approach to include all health services	Yes. Agreement to incorporate into strategy documents for future. No agreement on areas for disinvestment
Twaddle, Walker (1995)[5]	One Scottish Health Board	Gynaecology services	Yes. Agreement to incorporate findings into contracts
Craig, Parkin, Gerard (1995)[6]	One English HA	Macro approach to include all health services	No. Work ongoing
Brambleby (1995)[7]	Two localities within one English HA	All health services	Yes, in terms of communicating and informing. No in terms of changes implemented
Madden, Hussey, Mooney, Church (1995)[8]	Zonal agency, covering four HAs and three FHSAs in England	Two programmes: heart disease and mental health	No information provided
Street, Posnett, Davis (1995)[9]	One English HA	Dementia services	Yes. Expert group withdrew and the process was halted
Ratcliffe, Donaldson, Macphee (1996)[10]	One Scottish Health Board	Maternity services	No information provided
Ruta, Donaldson, Gilray (1996)[11]	One Scottish Health Board	Child health services	Yes. Recommendations from PBMA exercise incorporated into policy
Scott, Currie, Donaldson (1998)[12]	One Scottish Total Fundholding Pilot Site	Diabetes care	No information provided

References

1   Donaldson C and Farrar C (1993) Needs assessment: developing an economic approach. *Health Policy.* **25:** 95–108.

2   Cohen D (1994) Marginal analysis in practice: an alternative to needs assessment for contracting healthcare. *BMJ.* **309:** 781–5.

3   Cohen D (1995) Messages from Mid Glamorgan: a multi-programme experiment with marginal analysis. *Health Policy.* **33:** 147–55.

4   Lockett T, Raftery J and Richards J (1995) The strengths and limitations of programme budgeting. In: FR Honigsbaum and J Lockett (eds) *Priority Setting in Action.* Radcliffe Medical Press, Oxford.

5   Twaddle S and Walker A (1995) Programme budgeting and marginal analysis: application within programmes to assist purchasing in Greater Glasgow Health Board. *Health Policy.* **33:** 91–105.

6   Craig N, Parkin D and Gerard K (1995) Clearing the fog on the Tyne: programme budgeting in Newcastle and North Tyneside Health Authority. *Health Policy.* **33:** 107–25.

7   Brambleby P (1995) A survivor's guide to programme budgeting. *Health Policy.* **33:** 127–45.

8   Madden L *et al.* (1995) Public health and economics in tandem: programme budgeting, marginal analysis and priority setting in practice. *Health Policy.* **33:** 161–8.

9   Street APJ, Posnett J and Davis P (1995) *Marginal Analysis of Dementia Services.* Health Economics Consortium, University of York, York.

10 Ratcliffe J, Donaldson C and Macphee S (1996) Programme budgeting and marginal analysis: a case study of maternity services. *J Public Health Medicine.* **18(2):** 175–82.

11 Ruta D, Donaldson C and Gilray I (1996) Economics, public health and healthcare purchasing: the Tayside experience of programme budgeting and marginal analysis. *J Health Services Research Policy.* **1(4):** 185–93.

12 Scott A, Currie N and Donaldson C (1998) Evaluating innovation in general practice: a pragmatic framework using programme budgeting and marginal analysis. *Family Practice.* **15(3):** 216–22.

Index